AF762151

GERIATRICS, GERONTOLOGY AND ELDERLY ISSUES

NURSING HOMES AND ELDER ABUSE

GERIATRICS, GERONTOLOGY AND ELDERLY ISSUES

Additional books and e-books in this series can be found on Nova's website under the Series tab.

GERIATRICS, GERONTOLOGY AND ELDERLY ISSUES

NURSING HOMES AND ELDER ABUSE

JOSHUA NEWLAND
EDITOR

snova
New York

Copyright © 2020 by Nova Science Publishers, Inc.

All rights reserved. No part of this book may be reproduced, stored in a retrieval system or transmitted in any form or by any means: electronic, electrostatic, magnetic, tape, mechanical photocopying, recording or otherwise without the written permission of the Publisher.

We have partnered with Copyright Clearance Center to make it easy for you to obtain permissions to reuse content from this publication. Simply navigate to this publication's page on Nova's website and locate the "Get Permission" button below the title description. This button is linked directly to the title's permission page on copyright.com. Alternatively, you can visit copyright.com and search by title, ISBN, or ISSN.

For further questions about using the service on copyright.com, please contact:
Copyright Clearance Center
Phone: +1-(978) 750-8400 Fax: +1-(978) 750-4470 E-mail: info@copyright.com.

NOTICE TO THE READER

The Publisher has taken reasonable care in the preparation of this book, but makes no expressed or implied warranty of any kind and assumes no responsibility for any errors or omissions. No liability is assumed for incidental or consequential damages in connection with or arising out of information contained in this book. The Publisher shall not be liable for any special, consequential, or exemplary damages resulting, in whole or in part, from the readers' use of, or reliance upon, this material. Any parts of this book based on government reports are so indicated and copyright is claimed for those parts to the extent applicable to compilations of such works.

Independent verification should be sought for any data, advice or recommendations contained in this book. In addition, no responsibility is assumed by the Publisher for any injury and/or damage to persons or property arising from any methods, products, instructions, ideas or otherwise contained in this publication.

This publication is designed to provide accurate and authoritative information with regard to the subject matter covered herein. It is sold with the clear understanding that the Publisher is not engaged in rendering legal or any other professional services. If legal or any other expert assistance is required, the services of a competent person should be sought. FROM A DECLARATION OF PARTICIPANTS JOINTLY ADOPTED BY A COMMITTEE OF THE AMERICAN BAR ASSOCIATION AND A COMMITTEE OF PUBLISHERS.

Additional color graphics may be available in the e-book version of this book.

Library of Congress Cataloging-in-Publication Data

ISBN: 978-1-53617-974-3

Published by Nova Science Publishers, Inc. † New York

CONTENTS

PREFACE

Nursing homes provide care to about 1.4 million nursing home residents—a vulnerable population of elderly and disabled individuals. CMS, an agency within the Department of Health and Human Services (HHS), defines standards nursing homes must meet to participate in the Medicare and Medicaid programs. This book reviews the abuse of residents in nursing homes.

Chapter 1 - This is an edited, reformatted and augmented version of Hearing Before the Subcommittee on Oversight and Investigations of the Committee on Energy and Commerce House of Representatives, One Hundred fifteenth Congress, Second Session, Serial No. 115–164, dated September 6, 2018.

Chapter 2 - Nursing homes provide care to about 1.4 million nursing home residents—a vulnerable population of elderly and disabled individuals. CMS, an agency within the Department of Health and Human Services (HHS), defines standards nursing homes must meet to participate in the Medicare and Medicaid programs. GAO was asked to review abuse of residents in nursing homes. Among other objectives, this report: (1) determines the trends and types of abuse in recent years, and (2) evaluates CMS oversight intended to ensure residents are free from abuse. GAO reviewed CMS's policies, analyzed CMS data on abuse deficiencies from 2013 through 2017, the most recent data at the time of our review, and interviewed officials from CMS and state survey agencies in five states, as well as other key stakeholders in those states such as ombudsmen and law enforcement officials. The states were selected for variation in factors such as number of nursing homes and role of other state agencies in abuse investigations.

Chapter 3 - Nationwide, about 1.4 million elderly or disabled individuals receive care in more than 15,500 nursing homes. CMS, an agency within the Department of Health and Human Services (HHS), defines standards nursing homes must meet to participate in the Medicare and Medicaid programs. Nursing home residents often have physical or cognitive limitations that can leave them particularly vulnerable to abuse. Abuse of nursing home residents can occur in many forms—including physical, mental, verbal, and sexual— and can be committed by staff, residents, or others in the nursing home. Any incident of abuse is a serious occurrence and can result in potentially devastating consequences for residents, including lasting mental anguish, serious injury, or death. This statement summarizes GAO's June 2019 report, GAO-19-433. Specifically, it describes: (1) the trends and types of abuse in recent years, and (2) CMS's oversight intended to ensure residents are free from abuse. It also includes a brief summary of findings and recommendations from this June 2019 report and prior GAO reports that examined the health and welfare of the elderly in multiple settings, and the status, as of November 2019, of HHS's efforts to implement the recommendations GAO made.

Chapter 4 - The federal government and states share responsibility for the health and welfare of about 1.5 million individuals— most of them vulnerable older adults— receiving long-term care in nursing homes and assisted living facilities covered by Medicare and Medicaid. For nursing homes, which provide skilled nursing care, federal law defines applicable quality standards and CMS provides guidance for nursing homes and the state survey agencies to help protect residents from elder abuse. For assisted living facilities, which provide assistance with activities of daily living in a residential setting, CMS defines the framework states must establish to oversee these facilities if covered under Medicaid. This includes requiring states to demonstrate to CMS that they are assuring quality including the obligation to protect against elder abuse. GAO was asked to review federal oversight of elder abuse reporting, investigation, and law enforcement notification in both nursing homes and assisted living facilities. In this report, GAO describes federal requirements for reporting, investigating, and notifying law enforcement about elder abuse in both types of facilities. GAO reviewed relevant laws and regulations and agency guidance, and interviewed CMS and state officials from three states selected for variation in HCBS waiver program size and geography. GAO also interviewed representatives from national stakeholder groups representing consumers, facilities, Medicaid directors, and abuse investigators. In comments on this report, HHS highlighted the distinct oversight frameworks for the two settings and noted that CMS is undertaking efforts to strengthen oversight.

In: Nursing Homes and Elder Abuse
Editor: Joshua Newland
ISBN: 978-1-53617-974-3
© 2020 Nova Science Publishers, Inc.

Chapter 1

EXAMINING FEDERAL EFFORTS TO ENSURE QUALITY OF CARE AND RESIDENT SAFETY IN NURSING HOMES*

Committee on Energy and Commerce

Thursday, September 6, 2018
House of Representatives,
Subcommittee on Oversight and Investigations,
Committee on Energy and Commerce,
Washington, DC.

The subcommittee met, pursuant to call, at 10:15 a.m., in room 2322 Rayburn House Office Building, Hon. Gregg Harper (chairman of the subcommittee) presiding.

---

* This is an edited, reformatted and augmented version of Hearing Before the Subcommittee on Oversight and Investigations of the Committee on Energy and Commerce House of Representatives, One Hundred fifteenth Congress, Second Session, Serial No. 115–164, dated September 6, 2018.

Members present: Representatives Harper, Griffith, Burgess, Brooks, Walberg, Walters, Costello, Carter, Walden (ex officio), DeGette, Schakowsky, Castor, Clarke, Ruiz, and Pallone (ex officio).

Also present: Representative Bilirakis.

Staff present: Jennifer Barblan, Chief Counsel, Oversight and Investigations; Samantha Bopp, Staff Assistant; Lamar Echols, Counsel, Oversight and Investigations; Ali Fulling, Legislative Clerk, Oversight and Investigations, Digital Commerce and Consumer Protection; Christopher Santini, Counsel, Oversight and Investigations; Jennifer Sherman, Press Secretary; Julie Babayan, Minority Counsel; Jeff Carroll, Minority Staff Director; Tiffany Guarascio, Minority Deputy Staff Director and Chief Health Advisor; Chris Knauer, Minority Oversight Staff Director; Jourdan Lewis, Minority Staff Assistant and Policy Analyst; Kevin McAloon, Minority Professional Staff Member; and C.J. Young, Minority Press Secretary.

OPENING STATEMENT OF HON. GREGG HARPER, A REPRESENTATIVE IN CONGRESS FROM THE STATE OF MISSISSIPPI

Mr. HARPER. We will call to order today's subcommittee hearing, Oversight and Investigations, and our hearing today is on Examining Federal Efforts to Ensure Quality of Care and Resident Safety in Nursing Homes. I want to welcome each of our witnesses that are here today, and at this point I am going to recognize myself for our opening statement.

So this a very important subject and the subcommittee continues to work in examining whether the Federal Government is meeting its obligations to ensure that residents in nursing homes across the country are free from abuse and receiving the quality of care that they deserve and respect. Protecting our most vulnerable citizens is among the most fundamental responsibilities entrusted to the fFederal Government and it is also a responsibility that we as Americans all share.

The Centers for Medicare and Medicaid Services, CMS, is the Federal agency tasked with ensuring nursing home residents are protected and well cared for, and CMS largely relies on the efforts of State survey agencies to verify that nursing homes are meeting Federal standards for quality and safety.

However, reports issued by the Department of Health and Human Services Office of Inspector General and the Government Accountability Office, along with all too frequent press reports, detail horrible cases of abuse and neglect occurring in nursing homes raises questions as to whether CMS is fulfilling its obligations to residents. For example, in 2014, OIG found that based on its review of more than 650 medical records of Medicare beneficiaries that were receiving care in a nursing home, approximately one-third of residents experienced some type of harm during their stay. According to OIG, nearly 60 percent of this harm was either clearly preventable or likely preventable.

Last year, reports emerged out of Florida of the deaths of at least a dozen residents of the Rehabilitation Center at Hollywood Hills after the facility's air conditioning system failed in the immediate aftermath of Hurricane Irma. According to state regulators, temperatures at the facility reached nearly a hundred degrees and the facility deprived residents of timely medical care despite being located across the street from a fully functioning and functional hospital.

CMS described the events at this nursing home as a complete management failure and terminated the facility from the Medicare and Medicaid programs noting that the conditions at the facility constituted an immediate jeopardy to residents' health and safety. Previously, this facility's owner entered into a settlement agreement with the Federal Government to resolve allegations he and his associates had paid kickbacks and performed medically unnecessary treatments to generate Medicare and Medicaid payments at another Florida healthcare facility in which he had an ownership interest. Despite this history and last year's tragedy at that person's rehabilitation center, we have learned that the facility's owner continues to maintain an ownership interest in at least 11 facilities participating in the Medicare and Medicaid programs.

It can't be emphasized enough that it should not take a tragedy like what we have seen at the Rehabilitation Center at Hollywood Hills to make CMS mindful or take action in response of conditions at nursing homes that threaten residents' well-being. However, the committee's oversight and reports issued by OIG and GAO suggest that this isn't necessarily the case.

Improving care for vulnerable populations including the care provided to nursing home residents has been identified by OIG as a top management challenge for over a decade. We want to know why this continues to be a top management challenge, what steps CMS is taking to improve efforts to enforce existing regulatory requirements, and how the agency is addressing any gaps in its oversight.

At the same time, we want to recognize the many, and I mean many, nursing homes that are providing their residents with high quality care. In advance of this hearing I checked in with Vanessa Henderson, Executive Director for the Mississippi Health Care Association, for an update on our facilities after Tropical Storm Gordon made landfall late last night on the Mississippi Gulf Coast. Ms. Henderson received reports every 2 hours throughout the night from 19 nursing homes in nine South Mississippi counties. There were no major issues. They were well prepared.

When Hurricane Katrina devastated the Mississippi Gulf Coast, now 13 years ago, there was no fatality or major problem at a nursing home in Mississippi. And I am proud of these successes in my home State. What are the best practices being utilized at these facilities that if applied everywhere could yield positive outcomes for nursing home residents?

I look forward to hearing from each member on our panel on ways we can improve our Federal oversight of nursing homes to ensure that CMS is protecting seniors from abuse and neglect in nursing homes and using its authority in a fair and efficient manner. I thank you for your testimony today and I now recognize the ranking member of the subcommittee from Colorado, Ms. DeGette, for 5 minutes.

[The prepared statement of Mr. Harper follows:]

PREPARED STATEMENT OF HON. GREGG HARPER

Good morning, today the Subcommittee continues its work examining whether the federal government is meeting its obligations to ensure that residents in nursing homes across the country are free from abuse and are receiving the quality of care they deserve. Protecting our most vulnerable citizens is among the most fundamental responsibilities entrusted to the federal government, and it is also a responsibility that we, as Americans, all share.

The Centers for Medicare and Medicaid Services (CMS) is the federal agency tasked with ensuring nursing home residents are protected and well-cared for, and CMS largely relies on the efforts of state survey agencies to verify that nursing homes are meeting federal standards for quality and safety. However, reports issued by the Department of Health and Human Services' Office of Inspector General (OIG) and the Government Accountability Office (GAO), along with all too frequent press reports that detail horrible cases of abuse and neglect occurring in nursing homes, raise questions as to whether CMS is fulfilling its obligations to residents.

For example, in 2014 OIG found that, based on its review of more than 650 medical records of Medicare beneficiaries that were receiving care in a nursing home, approximately one-third of residents experienced some type of harm during their stay. According to OIG, nearly 60 percent of this harm was either clearly preventable or likely preventable.

Last year, reports emerged out of Florida of the deaths of at least a dozen residents of the Rehabilitation Center at Hollywood Hills after the facility's air conditioning system failed in the immediate aftermath of Hurricane Irma. According to state regulators, temperatures at the facility reached nearly 100 degrees and the facility deprived residents of timely medical care despite being located across the street from a fully-functional hospital. CMS described the events at this nursing home as a "complete management failure" and terminated the facility from the Medicare and Medicaid programs, noting the conditions at the facility constituted an immediate jeopardy to residents' health and safety.

Previously, the facility's owner entered into a settlement agreement with the federal government to resolve allegations he and his associates paid kickbacks and performed medically unnecessary treatments to generate Medicare and Medicaid payments at another Florida health care facility in which he had an ownership interest.

Despite this history, and last year's tragedy at the Rehabilitation Center, we have learned that the facility's owner continues to maintain an ownership interest in at least 11 facilities participating in the Medicare and Medicaid programs.

It can't be emphasized enough that it should not take a tragedy like what was seen at the Rehabilitation Center at Hollywood Hills to make CMS mindful, or take action in response, of conditions at nursing homes that threaten residents' well-being. However, the Committee's oversight, and reports issued by OIG and GAO, suggest that this isn't necessarily the case. Improving care for vulnerable populations, including the care provided to nursing home residents, has been identified by OIG as a top management challenge for over a decade. We want to know why this continues to be a top management challenge, what steps CMS is taking to improve efforts to enforce existing regulatory requirements, and how the agency is addressing any gaps in its oversight.

We also want to recognize the many nursing homes that are providing their residents with high quality care. In advance of this hearing, I checked in with Vanessa Henderson, Executive Director for the Mississippi Health Care Association, for an update on our facilities after Tropical Storm Gordon made landfall late last night on the Mississippi Gulf Coast.

Ms. Henderson received reports every two hours throughout the night from 19 nursing homes in 9 south Mississippi counties. There were no major issues. When Hurricane Katrina devastated the Mississippi Gulf Coast 13 years ago there was no fatality or major problem at a nursing home in Mississippi. I am proud of these successes in my home state. What are the best practices being utilized at these facilities that if applied elsewhere could yield positive outcomes for nursing home residents?

I look forward to hearing from each member of our panel on ways we can improve our federal oversight of nursing homes to ensure that CMS is protecting seniors from abuse and neglect in nursing homes and using its authorities in a fair and effective manner. I thank you for your testimony today and now recognize the Ranking Member of the Subcommittee from Colorado, Ms. DeGette, for five minutes.

OPENING STATEMENT OF HON. DIANA DEGETTE, A REPRESENTATIVE IN CONGRESS FROM THE STATE OF COLORADO

Ms. DeGette. Thank you so much, Mr. Chairman. I guess as proof that this subcommittee often, most often, works in a bipartisan way, my opening statement is pretty much exactly the same opening statement you just made down to the example of the Hollywood Hills tragedy after Hurricane Irma when 14 people died. So I am going to submit my written statement for the record, I just want to make a couple of observations.

The first one is some of us have been on this subcommittee for many, many years and those of you who have been here you know that for all of these years we have struggled to address the issue of quality care at nursing homes. Both the IG at HHS and also the GAO have consistently raised issues over the years about how the States and CMS oversee the nursing home industry and every so often we have a real tragedy like this Hollywood Hills tragedy.

But then, you have got to wonder how many more facilities are like this and what are we doing to make a permanent effort. It just seems like we haven't turned the corner to get where we need to be in providing effective oversight in this sector of care. For example, just today, the Inspector General in written testimony mentions a statistic that I find really troubling. Fully one-third of Medicare residents in a skilled nursing home experienced harm from the care that they received and half of those cases were actually preventable.

So we do this over and over again, but yet, one-third of Medicare residents have experienced harm. Now the IG has made recommendations for how to improve these issues. CMS needs to articulate to us today what concrete steps the agency is making to improve this. I also want to know what progress CMS is making on implementing the updated health and safety regulations that were finalized in 2016 after a lengthy rulemaking process.

It took years and a lot of public feedback, but in 2016 CMS did update the federal nursing home regulations to improve planning for resident care, training for staff, and protections against abuse, among other issues. But now as CMS is implementing these new rules, the agency has taken a series of actions that have led consumer groups, state attorneys general, and others to question whether CMS is doing enough to strengthen and enforce federal standards.

Here is a couple of examples: Last year CMS announced that it had imposed a moratorium on the enforcement of many of these regulations. In other words the agency is restraining itself from using some of its most effective enforcement tools against those who violate those new rules designed to protect vulnerable nursing home residents.

I must say CMS has to commit itself to implementing and enforcing its own regulations. That sounds kind of like a ridiculous thing to say but it is true, because as I said the core issue is here that frail and vulnerable people are harmed when nursing homes fail to meet our standards. And I don't think any of us wants to wait until the next natural disaster or other disaster exposes some kind of a deficiency that kills dozens of people.

I want to thank the witnesses for being here today. I want to thank the Inspector General and the GAO for your body of oversight of work on nursing homes, and I hope that we won't be back here again next year or in 5 years to talk about how more people have died. Thanks, and I yield back.

Mr. Harper. The gentlewoman yields back.

The chair will now recognize the gentleman from Oregon, the chairman of the full committee, Mr. Walden, for 5 minutes.

Opening Statement of Hon. Greg Walden, A Representative in Congress from the State of Oregon

Mr. Walden. Thank you very much, Mr. Chairman. Thanks for holding this hearing on this topic that is very important to all of us across the country.

I think it is important to put it all in context as well. According to information released by the Centers for Medicare and Medicaid Services, more than three million individuals rely on services provided by nursing homes at some point during every year. And on any given day, 1.4 million Americans reside in more than 15,000 nursing homes across our country and the overwhelming majority of these nursing homes provide high quality, lifesaving care to their residents. We know that too.

I have heard from many seniors and their families in my district about how they or their loved ones are receiving excellent, around- the-clock care at their nursing homes and they go above and beyond. One provider I spoke with recently has a facility down in Redding, California. And when the fires were threatening Redding he chartered buses, had them on the ready with 200 seats, made arrangements, and all of this was happening very, very quickly to be able to move patients, residents to a facility many miles away in Klamath Falls, Oregon, if need be. As it turned out he didn't have to do that evacuation, but they were ready. Unfortunately, this doesn't appear to be the case in all nursing homes.

We all know the discussion that has occurred around what happened at the Rehabilitation Center at Hollywood Hills, Florida, run by Dr. Jack Michel. That tragedy that occurred at that facility during Hurricane Irma was the result of inexcusable management or mismanagement and it resulted in needless loss of life.

While many facilities in Florida had the right procedures in place and handled the hurricanes well, we need to make sure our Federal oversight efforts are effective in detecting low quality, unsafe nursing homes while being mindful to not impose excessive regulatory burdens that in some cases don't help but cost a lot of money and tie up resources. So I think we need to look at that as well, what is working and what is not, to get to the underlying problems we have identified in the OIG and others have.

As Chairman Harper described, CMS is the Federal agency responsible for ensuring the safety and quality of care provided to Medicare and Medicaid beneficiaries in nursing homes. CMS enters into these agreements with the states providing that state agencies will inspect nursing homes on CMS' behalf to determine whether the facilities are meeting Federal requirements.

And so this is done by the states. However, CMS may not always be effectively overseeing that work that these agencies do on behalf of the federal government. Over the last decade or so, the Department of Health and Human Services Office of Inspector General and Government Accountability Office have both issued reports indicating CMS could improve its oversight of nursing homes.

For example, HHS OIG has examined whether States properly verify that deficiencies identified during nursing home inspections are corrected. In some instances, such as my State of Oregon, HHS OIG found the State properly verified that facilities corrected deficiencies after they were identified and during inspections.

Several of the reports on this topic, however, HHS OIG has found that state agencies elsewhere did not meet that standard of proper oversight. For example, a report issued this May estimated that in 2016 Nebraska failed to properly verify that deficiencies at nursing homes identified during state inspections were corrected 92 percent of the time. CMS needs to ensure that all state survey agencies are adequately conducting the survey process on their behalf.

We are looking forward to hearing what CMS is doing to improve its oversight of the survey process. We also look forward to hearing from GAO about their work and recommendations, especially their recommendations relating to CMS' oversight of state survey agencies. So the focus of today's hearing is to learn more about what CMS is doing to maintain consistency across the country and guarantee that all States are effectively surveying nursing homes on their behalf to ensure compliance with existing Federal requirements.

We also want to know what we can do to help in these efforts. So it is important that CMS effectively enforce existing requirements for nursing homes to protect and promote safety, especially in extreme cases like what happened at the Rehabilitation Center at Hollywood Hills. And lastly, I want to thank our witnesses for being a part of this important conversation. We very much value and appreciate your testimony.

With that Mr. Chair, unless anyone else wants the remainder— Dr. Burgess chairs our Subcommittee on Health—I yield the balance to you.

[The prepared statement of Mr. Walden follows:]

PREPARED STATEMENT OF HON. GREG WALDEN

Thank you, Mr. Chairman, for holding this hearing on the very important issue of protecting one of the most vulnerable populations in the United States— the elderly.

According to information released by the Centers for Medicare and Medicaid Services (CMS), more than three million individuals rely on services provided by nursing homes at some point during the year. On any given day, 1.4 million Americans reside in the more than 15,000 nursing homes across our country. The overwhelming majority of these nursing homes provide high quality, life-saving care to their residents.

I've heard from many seniors and their families in my district about how they or their loved ones are receiving excellent, around the clock care at their nursing homes. And many go above and beyond.

One provider I spoke with recently has a facility in Redding, California, and set a good example of what to strive for in preparing for an emergency, with 200 seats on buses ready to go at a moment's notice, and agreements with providers in Klamath Falls, Oregon to house their patients if this summer's devastating wildfires threatened their facility.

Unfortunately, this doesn't appear to be the case in all nursing homes across the country, such as the Rehabilitation Center in Hollywood Hills, Florida, run by Dr. Jack Michel. The tragedy that occurred at this facility during Hurricane Irma was a result of inexcusable management, and it resulted in needless loss of life. While many facilities in Florida had the right procedures in place and handled the hurricanes well, we need to make sure our federal oversight efforts are effective in detecting low quality, unsafe nursing homes while being mindful to not to impose excessive regulatory burdens that, in some cases, may actually hinder resident care.

As Chairman Harper described, CMS is the federal agency responsible for ensuring the safety and quality of care provided to Medicare and Medicaid beneficiaries in nursing homes. CMS enters into agreements with individual states, providing that state agencies will inspect nursing homes on CMS' behalf to determine whether the facilities in a particular state meet federal requirements to participate in these programs.

However, CMS may not always be effectively overseeing the work that these state agencies are doing on its behalf. Over the last decade or so, the Department of Health and Human Services' (HHS) Office of Inspector General (OIG) and the Government Accountability Office (GAO) have both issued reports indicating that CMS could improve its oversight of nursing homes.

For example, HHS OIG has examined whether states properly verify that deficiencies identified during nursing home inspections are corrected. In some instances, such as my home state of Oregon, HHS OIG has found that the state properly verified that facilities corrected deficiencies after they were identified during inspections. In several of the reports on this topic, however, HHS OIG has found that state agencies did not meet that standard of proper oversight. For example, a report issued this past May, estimated that in 2016 Nebraska failed to properly verify that deficiencies at nursing homes identified during state inspections were corrected 92 percent of the time. CMS needs to ensure that all state survey agencies are adequately conducting the survey process on their behalf. We are looking forward to hearing what CMS is doing to improve its oversight of the survey process.

We also look forward to hearing from GAO about their work and recommendations – especially their recommendations relating to CMS' oversight of state survey agencies.

The focus of today's hearing is to learn more about what CMS is doing to maintain consistency across the country and guarantee that all states are effectively surveying nursing homes on their behalf to ensure compliance with existing federal requirements. We also want to know what we can do to help these efforts.

It is important that CMS effectively enforce existing requirements for nursing homes to protect and promote patient safety, especially in extreme cases like what happened at the Rehabilitation Center at Hollywood Hills. Lastly, I'd like to thank our witnesses for being a part of this important conversation and look forward to their testimony.

Mr. Burgess. Well, thank you, Chairman Walden.

And I just want to mention that like Representative DeGette, in January of 2006 this subcommittee held a hearing, field hearing, in New Orleans, Louisiana, dealing with just this issue. So this morning it is important to see not just one of the lessons learned but how it is the implementation of those lessons and how really report not just to us, on us, how we are doing in overseeing the oversight that the agency is supposed to provide to the facilities that are taking care of our seniors.

So thank you, Mr. Chairman, for doing this hearing and I will yield back.

Mr. Harper. The gentleman yields back.

The chair will now recognize the ranking member of the full committee, Mr. Pallone, for 5 minutes.

OPENING STATEMENT OF HON. FRANK PALLONE, JR., A REPRESENTATIVE IN CONGRESS FROM THE STATE OF NEW JERSEY

Mr. PALLONE. Thank you, Mr. Chairman. Nursing home residents are among our most vulnerable populations who are often unable to care for themselves and require personal attention. Many of us have had loved ones in the care of nursing homes or skilled nursing facilities so we can all appreciate the need to ensure these facilities are providing high quality care. Most of the time nursing homes are staffed by compassionate professionals who want to provide quality care to those who need it and these professionals are strong allies too in our efforts to ensure residents are properly taken care of.

As the Department of Health and Human Services Office of Inspector General points out in his testimony today, nursing homes offer enormous benefit by providing a place of comfort and healing to residents in fragile health, many of whom are insured by Medicaid. The best nursing homes provide excellent care and take seriously their duty to protect their residents.

That said, nursing home quality of care is a longstanding concern and we should always strive to conduct oversight of this sector in an effort to improve the overall quality of care. And over the past several years, HHS's OIG and the Government Accountability Office have both found problems in nursing home delivery of care and Federal and State oversight. And that is not to say that we should be suspicious of all nursing homes, rather, certain providers have failed to ensure high quality care.

For example, OIG has found that when incidents of abuse or neglect occur some nursing homes fail to report them as required and GAO has identified gaps in nursing homes' emergency preparedness and response capabilities. We can and must demand better for our loved ones and that is why we must focus our resources to weed out these bad actors so that residents are protected and the rest of the industry is not given a black eye.

And that is where the Centers for Medicare and Medicaid Services comes in. In exchange for participating in the Medicare/Medicaid programs, nursing homes must comply with Federal standards related to health and safety. CMS is charged with overseeing nursing homes' compliance with those standards and the agency has enforcement mechanisms at its disposal. And among those standards are the ability to terminate a facility participation in Medicare and Medicaid if it does not comply, however, OIG and GAO have long raised questions about CMS' oversight of nursing homes.

For instance, OIG notes that CMS does not always ensure that abuse and neglect at skilled nursing facilities are identified and reported, and when a nursing home is cited for deficiency OIG has found that CMS does not always require them to correct the problem. Many of these same issues have been raised for several years so the committee needs to hear what progress CMS is making and what more needs to be done to better ensure quality of care.

CMS also relies on state survey agencies to conduct inspections of nursing homes on CMS' behalf, but some States have been better than others at ensuring high quality care. OIG's audits have revealed that several States fell short in investigating the most serious complaints and many had difficulty meeting CMS' standards. Workforce shortages and inexperienced surveyors at the state level have also led to the understatement of serious care problems. And, hereto, OIG and GAO have found problems with CMS' oversight of the state agencies. We need to hear what CMS needs to do better or differently to ensure Federal requirements are being followed.

And, finally, CMS has yet to finalize and enforce some 2016 regulations to update and strengthen the nursing home standards. These regulations address critical areas such as staff training and protections against abuse, among other issues. However, last year, CMS issued a moratorium on enforcement of many of these regulations. And it is important to hear the input of industry and consumer groups to ensure regulations are done right, but without actually enforcing these rules it is unclear how CMS will ensure the quality and safety of our nation's nursing homes.

So Dr. Goodrich needs to articulate today how CMS is considering the concerns of the industry and consumers while also meeting its responsibility to ensure high quality care in nursing homes. I yield back, Mr., I mean unless anybody else wants the time, but I don't think so. I yield back.

Mr. Harper. The gentleman yields back. I ask unanimous consent that the members' written opening statements be made part of the record. Without objection, they will so be entered into the record. I also ask unanimous consent that members of the full committee on Energy and

Commerce not on this subcommittee be permitted to participate in today's hearing.

I would now like to introduce our witnesses for today's hearing. Today we have Dr. Kate Goodrich, the Director of the Center for Clinical Standards and Quality, and Chief Medical Officer at the Centers for Medicare and Medicaid Services. We welcome you today.

Next is Ms. Ruth Ann Dorrill, Regional Inspector General at the Office of Inspector General at the U.S. Department of Health and Human Services. Thank you for being here today.

And, finally, Mr. John Dicken, Director of Health Care at the U.S. Government Accountability Office.

You are each aware that this committee is holding an investigative hearing and when doing so has had the practice of taking testimony under oath. Do you have any objection to testifying under oath?

Let the record reflect that all three have indicated no. The chair then advises you that under the rules of the House and the rules of the committee you are entitled to be accompanied by counsel. Do you desire to be accompanied by counsel during your testimony today?

All of the witnesses have indicated no.

In that case if you would please stand and raise your right hand, I will swear you in.

[Witnesses sworn.]

Mr. Harper. Thank you. You may be seated. You are now under oath and subject to the penalties set forth in Title 18 Section 1001 of the United States Code. You may now give a 5-minute summary of your written testimony.

And we will begin with you, Dr. Goodrich, and you are recognized for 5. We would ask that you pull the microphone a little closer to you and make sure that the mic is on. And you know the light system is such when it gets to yellow you have 1 minute. Red, the floor will not open up, but do bring it in for a landing, OK. Thank you.

You may begin.

STATEMENT OF KATE GOODRICH

Dr. Goodrich. All right. To Chairman Harper, Ranking Member DeGette, and members of the subcommittee, thank you for the opportunity to discuss CMS' efforts to oversee nursing homes.

Resident safety is our top priority in nursing homes and all facilities that participate in the Medicare and Medicaid programs. Every nursing home must keep its residents safe and provide high quality care. Monitoring patient safety and quality of care in nursing homes requires coordinated efforts between the Federal Government and the States.

To participate in Medicare or Medicaid, a nursing home must be certified as meeting numerous statutory and regulatory requirements including those pertaining the health, safety and quality. Compliance with these requirements for participation is verified through annual unannounced, onsite surveys conducted by state survey agencies in each of the 50 States, the District of Columbia, and the U.S. territories. When a state surveyor finds a serious violation of Federal regulation they report it to CMS and swift action is taken.

In cases of immediate jeopardy, meaning a facility's noncompliance has caused or is likely to cause serious injury, harm, or even death we can terminate the facility's participation agreement within as little as 2 days. Civil monetary penalties can also be assessed up to approximately $20,000 per day or per instance until substantial compliance is achieved. Other remedies could include in-service training or denial of payments.

For deficiencies that do not constitute immediate jeopardy, these deficiencies must be corrected within 6 months or the facility will be terminated from the program. Facilities are also required by law to report any allegation of abuse or neglect to their state survey agency and other appropriate authorities such as law enforcement or adult protective services.

When CMS learns that a nursing home has failed to report or investigate instances of abuse we take immediate action. For example, CMS issued a civil monetary penalty of almost $350,000 to one nursing home when a state surveyor found they did not properly investigate or prevent additional abuse involving eight residents.

We are always taking steps to enhance our quality and safety oversight efforts. Last fall, surveyors began verifying facility compliance with CMS' updated and improved emergency preparedness requirements. Facilities are now required to address location-specific hazards and responses, must have emergency or standby power systems and ensure they are operational during an emergency, develop additional staff training, and implement a communications system to contact necessary persons regarding resident care and health status in a timely manner.

In addition, in 2016, CMS updated the nursing home requirements to reflect the substantial advances into theory and practice of service delivery that have been made since 1991 such as ensuring that nursing home staff are properly trained in caring for residents with dementia. Given the number of revisions, CMS has provided a phased-in approach for facilities to meet these new requirements. We are in the second of three implementation phases and we are taking a thoughtful approach to implementation and providing education to providers while holding them accountable for any deficiencies.

Promoting transparency is another key factor to incentivizing quality. By using a five-star quality rating system, our Nursing Home Compare website provides residents and their families with an easy way to understand meaningful distinctions between high and low performing facilities on three factors: health inspections, quality measures, and staffing. In April of this year, we took steps to make staffing data more accurate. The new payroll-based journal data provide unprecedented insight into how facilities are staffed which can be used to analyze how facility staffing relates to quality and patient outcomes.

Under the new systems, facilities reporting 7 or more days in a quarter with no registered nurse hours or whose audits identify significant inaccuracies between the hours reported and the hours verified will receive a one-star staffing rating which will reduce the facility's overall rating by one star.

CMS greatly appreciates and relies on the work of the Government Accountability Office and the HHS Office of the Inspector General to inform our efforts. We have implemented a number of recommendations in this area and we look forward to additional recommendations to help us continuously improve our programs.

For example, CMS implemented a new survey process last fall that provides standardization and structure to help ensure consistency between surveyors while allowing surveyors the autonomy to make decisions based upon their expertise and judgment. We expect every nursing home to keep its residents safe and provide high quality care. As a practicing physician that makes rounds in the hospital on weekends, many of my patients are frail, elderly nursing home residents, so I am personally deeply committed to the care of these patients.

CMS remains diligent in its duties to monitor nursing homes participating in the Medicare and Medicaid programs across the country and we look forward to continuing to work with Congress, States, facilities, residents, and other stakeholders to make sure the residents we serve are receiving safe and high quality care. I look forward to answering questions you may have. Thank you.

[The prepared statement of Dr. Goodrich follows:]

STATEMENT OF

KATE GOODRICH, M.D.,

DIRECTOR,

CENTER FOR CLINICAL STANDARDS AND QUALITY, AND

CHIEF MEDICAL OFFICER,

CENTERS FOR MEDICARE & MEDICAID SERVICES

ON

"EXAMING FEDERAL EFFORTS TO ENSURE QUALITY OF CARE AND RESIDENT SAFETY IN NURSING HOMES"

BEFORE THE

U. S. HOUSE ENERGY AND COMMERCE COMMITTEE,
SUBCOMMITTEE ON OVERSIGHT AND INVESTIGATIONS

SEPTEMBER 6, 2018

U. S. House Energy and Commerce Committee,
Subcommittee on Oversight and Investigations
"Examining Federal Efforts to Ensure Quality of Care and Resident Safety in Nursing Homes"
September 6, 2018

Chairman Harper, Ranking Member DeGette, and members of the Subcommittee, thank you for the invitation and the opportunity to discuss efforts at the Centers for Medicare & Medicaid Services (CMS) to oversee nursing homes. Resident safety is our top priority. It is the duty of every nursing home serving Medicare and Medicaid residents to keep its residents safe and provide high quality care.

Monitoring patient safety and quality of care in nursing homes serving Medicare and Medicaid beneficiaries requires coordinated efforts between the federal government and the states. To qualify for payment for services to beneficiaries, a nursing home must be enrolled in and certified by CMS as a skilled nursing facility under the Medicare program or a nursing facility under the Medicaid program. States play a critical role in helping CMS survey for facility compliance with both federal and state requirements, such as licensure.

To become certified as a Medicare and Medicaid participating provider of services, a nursing home must meet federal statutory and regulatory requirements which include a list of specific requirements for participation pertaining to health, safety and quality.[1] Compliance with these requirements for participation is verified through unannounced on-site surveys. Nursing homes must remain in substantial compliance with these requirements, as well as state law, to continue as a Medicare or Medicaid participating provider. Our efforts are informed and improved by the work of the Government Accountability Office (GAO) and the Department of Health and Human Services Office of Inspector General (HHS-OIG), and we greatly appreciate their recommendations and ongoing assistance to ensure resident safety and facility compliance.

---

[1] Sections 1819 and 1919 of the Social Security Act and 42 C.F.R. Parts 483 and 489.

In addition to these quality and safety oversight efforts, CMS has made improving the quality of care provided in nursing homes and providing information to consumers about nursing home quality a top priority. For example, in response to quality and safety concerns related to the use of antipsychotic medications among a growing number of residents with dementia, CMS launched the National Partnership to Improve Dementia Care in Nursing Homes, which has worked to optimize the quality of care and quality of life for residents in America's nursing homes by improving care for all residents, especially those with dementia, by reducing the use of antipsychotic medications and enhancing the use of nonpharmacologic approaches and person-centered dementia care practices. The CMS Nursing Home Compare[2] website provides detailed information for comparison of nursing homes and features a Five-Star Quality Rating System to help consumers, their families, and caregivers compare nursing homes more easily. At the direction of Administrator Seema Verma, CMS has been working tirelessly to evaluate and streamline regulations and operations with the goal to reduce unnecessary burden, increase efficiencies, and improve the customer experience for nursing facilities so that the priority is the care of the patient.

Quality and Safety Oversight

CMS works with state survey agencies in each of the 50 states, the District of Columbia, Puerto Rico, and other U.S. territories to perform surveys of providers and suppliers. For nursing homes, state survey agencies inspect these providers for compliance with Medicare and Medicaid health and safety standards related to both delivery and monitoring of care, as well as Life Safety Code requirements intended to protect residents by providing a reasonable degree of safety from fire. The states also take intake of complaints and conduct investigations accordingly.

[2] Available at: https://www.medicare.gov/nursinghomecompare/search.html

Facilities must meet state licensure requirements, in addition to CMS statutory and regulatory requirements, to be certified as a Medicare and Medicaid provider. The state survey agency, working on behalf of CMS, is usually the same agency responsible for both state licensure and Federal surveys and oversight. Therefore, these on-site surveys are often performed by the same state team at the same time, with the findings entered into two separate survey reports: one for state licensure purposes and one for Medicare and Medicaid compliance purposes. Utilizing the expertise of state officials to perform surveys means that state agencies and officials have up-to-date information on health and safety risks at facilities, and, as appropriate, can take direct action against facilities through state licensure sanction as well as recommend federal enforcement actions and remedies in response to deficiencies with health and safety requirements.

CMS is always looking for ways to improve our quality and safety oversight efforts to safeguard nursing home residents. CMS recently updated and improved the emergency preparedness requirements for nursing homes and other providers participating in Medicare and Medicaid.[3] For example, we clarified that certified nursing homes must have emergency electrical power systems for lighting entrances and doorways and maintaining fire detection, alarm, extinguishing systems as well as life support systems, must have emergency and stand-by-power systems and have a plan for ensuring these systems are operational during an emergency, and introduced additional testing requirements for these emergency and stand-by-power systems. In addition, we required facilities to develop an emergency preparedness training and testing program for new and existing staff, contracted service providers, and volunteers, as well as periodic refresher training. Facilities were required to comply with the new emergency preparedness on November 15, 2016, and surveys to evaluate compliance with the new requirements began on November 15, 2017.

CMS also made revisions to the other nursing home requirements in late 2016. These changes reflect the first comprehensive review and update

---

[3] https://www.federalregister.gov/documents/2016/09/16/2016-21404/medicare-and-medicaid-programs-emergency- preparedness-requirements-for-medicare-and-medicaid

of the regulations since 1991. These updated regulations reflect the substantial advances that have been made over the past several years in theory and practice of service delivery and safety and address important public health priorities such as combatting multi-drug resistant organisms among this vulnerable population. The changes made to the regulations include ensuring nursing home staff are properly trained on caring for residents with dementia and in preventing elder abuse, facilities take into consideration the health of residents when making decisions on the kinds and level of staffing a facility needs, staff have the right skills and competencies to provide person-centered care, resident's care plans take into consideration goals of cares and preferences, improvements to care planning including discharge planning, allowing dieticians and therapy providers the authority to write orders when delegated by a physician and state licensing laws allow, and updating the infection and control program including requiring an infection prevention and control officer and an antibiotic stewardship program. These revisions are also an integral part of our efforts to achieve broad improvements both in the quality of health care furnished through federal programs, and in patient safety, while at the same time reducing procedural burdens on providers.

Given the number of revised and new requirements in this rule, CMS is implementing it in three phases. The three phases were determined based on complexity of the revisions and the work necessary to revise the interpretive guidance and survey process based on the revisions. The requirements under Phase 1 implemented in November 2016, included those that did not impose additional requirements on facilities or were straightforward to implement. Phase 2 requirements are new requirements and those provisions that required more complex revisions; these were implemented in November 2017. CMS also implemented a revised survey process at this time to strengthen the survey system incorporating these new requirements. On November 24, 2017, CMS announced a temporary moratorium on the imposition of certain enforcement remedies such as civil monetary penalties for eight Phase 2 requirements, because of concerns from stakeholders about the scope and timing of their implementation.[4] CMS is using this 18-month moratorium period to educate nursing homes and providers to ensure they understand the health and safety expectations that will be evaluated through the survey process. However, the Phase 2 temporary moratorium is limited to 8 of 194 requirements and does not include those deficiencies related to abuse or neglect of residents. It also does not pause those enforcement activities that are required by federal law such as termination for immediate jeopardy findings that are not resolved. Compliance with all Phase 2 requirements is still monitored and cited, which is reflected in facilities' survey reports. In addition, all deficiencies are required by federal law to be corrected within 6 months or the facility will be terminated from participating in the Medicare and Medicaid programs.

Nursing homes are required by law to receive a recertification survey on an annual basis. Generally, state survey agencies conduct nursing home recertification surveys every year on behalf of CMS to assess facility compliance. However, complaint surveys can be performed at any time, with the actual timing dependent on the severity of the allegation. The Nursing Home Compare website includes links and other helpful information to help patients and families determine when and how to file a complaint.[5] In addition, nursing homes are required to post similar information on how to file complaints and grievances in their facilities.

When state inspectors identify violations of federal certification requirements, they notify the facility and in serious cases refer the case to CMS for enforcement. In most cases, the facility is required to develop a plan of correction to address identified violations within a time period depending on the scope and severity of the noncompliance violation. Enforcement actions where administrative remedies are imposed are taken against nursing homes that are not in compliance with Federal requirements. The law provides that CMS or the state authority impose one or more remedies when a facility is found to be out of substantial compliance with Federal requirements. When immediate jeopardy to

---

[4] https://www.cms.gov/Medicare/Provider-Enrollment-and- Certification/ SurveyCertificationGenInfo/Downloads/Survey-and-Cert-Letter-18-04.pdf

[5] https://www.medicare.gov/NursingHomeCompare/Resources/State-Websites.html

resident health and safety exists (meaning that the facility's noncompliance with one or more requirements has caused, or is likely to cause, serious injury, harm, impairment, or death), a CMS Regional Office or state Medicaid agency must take immediate action to remove the jeopardy and correct the deficiency by either terminating the facility or installing temporary management in as few as two calendar days after the facility receives notice that immediate jeopardy exists. Civil monetary penalties can also be assessed up to approximately $20,000 per day (or per instance) until substantial compliance is achieved for the deficiency identified. For deficiencies that do not constitute immediate jeopardy, remedies could include directed in-service training, denial of payments, or civil monetary penalties. Termination of a facility's Medicare and Medicaid participation is required by law for nursing homes that do not achieve substantial compliance for non-immediate jeopardy deficiencies within six months.

For those nursing homes which have more deficiencies than average, more serious deficiencies, or a pattern of serious deficiencies persisting over a long period of time, CMS may designate the nursing home as a Special Focus Facility[6], which requires the nursing home to be visited in person by survey teams twice as frequently as other nursing homes. CMS has strengthened the Special Focus Facility, or SFF, program over the past several years to ensure that homes either improve so that they can graduate from the program or they are terminated from Medicare/Medicaid participation. The longer the problems persist, the more stringent we are in the enforcement actions that will be taken. The objective of all remedies is to incentivize swift and sustained compliance in order to protect resident health and safety. Within about 18-24 months after a facility is identified by CMS as an SFF nursing home, we expect that the facility would improve and graduate from this program, be terminated from the Medicare or Medicaid program, or show progress but continue as an SFF nursing home for some additional time.

CMS is dedicated to maintaining an enforcement system that is centered on promoting high quality resident-centered health and safety for

[6] For more information see: https://www.cms.gov/Medicare/Provider-Enrollment-and-Certification/CertificationandComplianc/downloads/SFFList.pdf

nursing home residents. It is always our goal to ensure patient access to care while making sure patients are safe and appropriately cared for. CMS collaborates with state partners to educate nursing homes regarding our requirements, making sure they have the information they need to address any violations found during a survey. It is our hope that our efforts will help facilities come back into compliance, as well as prevent future noncompliance, without requiring termination from the Medicare and Medicaid programs. Nevertheless, we will terminate facilities that do not appropriately correct deficiencies because it is our obligation to ensure all nursing home facilities are safe and can meet resident needs.

CMS also leads the National Nursing Home Quality Care Collaborative with the Quality Innovation Network-Quality Improvement Organizations. The Collaborative launched in April 2015 with the mission to improve care for the 1.4 million nursing home residents across the country. The Collaborative works to rapidly spread the practices of high performing nursing homes to every nursing home in the country with the aim of ensuring that every nursing home resident receives the highest quality of care. Specifically, the Collaborative strives to instill quality and performance improvement practices, eliminate healthcare-acquired conditions, and dramatically improve resident satisfaction by focusing on the systems that impact quality, such as staffing, operations, communication, leadership, compliance, clinical models, quality of life indicators, and specific, clinical outcomes. Every state in the country has a significant percentage of nursing homes that voluntarily participate in this collaborative.

CMS also works with GAO and HHS-OIG to identify problems and implement recommendations that can improve our oversight of nursing home facilities. For example, GAO recommended that CMS develop timeframes and milestones for the development and implementation of a standardized survey methodology across all states.[7] CMS has implemented a new computer-based standardized survey process for nursing homes that is resident-centered which emphasizes evidence of potential quality of care issues and concerns identified through resident observation and interviews.

---

[7] See: https://www.gao.gov/assets/680/673480.pdf

This new survey process provides additional standardization and structure to help ensure consistency between surveyors while allowing surveyors the autonomy to make decisions based on their expertise and judgment.

Addressing Suspected Abuse and Neglect in Nursing Homes

Abuse and mistreatment of nursing home residents is never permitted, and CMS takes any allegation of these types of incidents very seriously. CMS requires nursing homes to report allegations of abuse and neglect immediately to their State Survey Agencies. When we learn a nursing home failed to report or investigate incidents of abuse, CMS takes immediate action against the nursing home. For example, in 2017, when a state surveyor found that a nursing home did not properly investigate or prevent additional abuse involving 8 residents, the nursing home was cited with noncompliance at the most serious immediate jeopardy level and was assessed a civil monetary penalty totaling approximately $347,000. In addition to issuing civil monetary penalties, CMS can deny payments or terminate a facility's Medicare and Medicaid participation agreements when appropriate. Since November 2017, CMS has issued noncompliance deficiency citations for nursing homes for failure to report or investigate allegations of abuse or neglect 2,323 times.

Section 1150B of the Social Security Act requires covered individuals such as employees, contractors and operators of federally funded nursing homes to report immediately to the HHS Secretary and local law enforcement any reasonable suspicion of a crime (as defined by local law enforcement) committed against a resident of a nursing home. CMS has taken a number of steps to implement the reporting requirements under section 1150B of the Social Security Act since enactment of this provision. CMS has issued memoranda, developed education tools for nursing facility staff, and provided outreach to State Survey Agencies regarding these requirements. Specifically, in 2011, CMS issued memoranda[8] informing

---

[8]https://www.cms.gov/Medicare/Provider-Enrollment-and-Certification/SurveyCertificationGenInfo/Downloads/SCLetter11_30.pdf

nursing homes of these new reporting requirements and the process for dealing with reporting of suspected crimes. In 2012, we developed a toolkit[9] that addressed abuse and the section 1150B reporting requirements and mailed this training program to all nursing facilities in the country. In 2016, section 1150B requirements were formally incorporated into federal regulations through notice and comment rulemaking. In 2017, CMS published sub-regulatory guidance that provided further clarification these requirements.[10] Specifically, this guidance clarifies terms in the regulation such as "reasonable suspicion of a crime" and describes the process the State Survey Agency uses to evaluate compliance with the requirements. CMS also released training information related to the reporting requirements, including a video that trains surveyors and the public on the minimum facility requirements in preventing abuse and neglect of nursing home residents. The state surveyors began surveying nursing facilities specifically regarding the 1150B requirements on November 28, 2017.

Additionally, CMS has been coordinating with HHS-OIG regarding the formal delegation of the authority to impose a civil monetary penalty against individuals covered under section 1150B and the facility for retaliation against such individuals, and the authority to permissively exclude those same individuals, as well as the noncompliant facilities, from any federal health care programs. The OIG currently has similar enforcement authorities under sections 1128 and 1128A of the Social Security Act.

We anticipate that this formal delegation will be completed shortly. However, irrespective of the formal delegation, because a nursing home's obligations under section 1150B have been incorporated into program participation requirements, if an instance of noncompliance with these requirements by facilities were to be identified, enforcement sanctions such as civil monetary penalties, denial of payments, and termination of a facility's Medicare and Medicaid participation agreements, can be imposed under CMS's existing enforcement authority under sections 1819(h) and

[9] https://surveyortraining.cms.hhs.gov/pubs/ClassInformation.aspx?cid=0CMSHANDINHAND

[10] https://www.cms.gov/Medicare/Provider-Enrollment-and-Certification/GuidanceforLawsAndRegulations/Nursing- Homes.html

1919(h) of the Act. CMS will continue to work with the HHS-OIG to enhance our ability to hold covered individuals accountable for reporting in addition to facilities as a whole and intend to issue regulations regarding enforcement following the formal delegation.

While CMS is not a law enforcement agency, we take cases of patient neglect and abuse very seriously and we work with state agencies, law enforcement, nursing home leadership and staff to ensure this vulnerable population is properly cared for and that all viable or alleged instances involving abuse or neglect are fully investigated and resolved. We are always looking to improve our programs and find better ways to identify, track, and, most importantly, prevent cases of neglect or abuse. To improve our current enforcement efforts, we will continue to work in partnership with GAO, HHS OIG, Congress, Regional Offices, states, consumer advocates, national associations, and other stakeholders.

National Partnership to Improve Dementia Care in Nursing Homes

Through our the National Partnership to Improve Dementia Care in Nursing Homes[11] (National Partnership), CMS has partnered with federal and state agencies, nursing homes, other providers, advocacy groups, and caregivers to improve comprehensive dementia care. CMS and our partners are committed to finding new ways to implement practices that enhance the quality of life for people with dementia, protect them from substandard care and promote goal-directed, person-centered care for every nursing home resident. The Partnership promotes a multidimensional approach that includes public reporting, state-based coalitions, research, training, and revised surveyor guidance. While the initial focus of the partnership was on reducing the use of antipsychotic medications, the larger mission is to

---

[11] https://www.cms.gov/Medicare/Provider-Enrollment-and-Certification/SurveyCertificationGenInfo/National- Partnership-to-Improve-Dementia-Care-in-Nursing-Homes.html

enhance the use of nonpharmacologic approaches and person-centered dementia care practices.

Since the launch of the National Partnership, significant reductions in the prevalence of antipsychotic medication use in long-stay nursing home residents have been documented. Between the end of 2011 and the end of quarter one of 2017, the national prevalence of antipsychotic use in long-stay nursing home residents was reduced by 34.1 percent, decreasing from 23.9 percent to 15.7 percent nationwide. All 50 states showed improvement with some states showing much more improvement than others. The National Partnership continues to work with state coalitions and nursing homes to reduce that rate even further. In October 2017, CMS announced a new national goal, involving a 15 percent reduction of antipsychotic medication use by the end of 2019[12] for long-stay residents in those homes with currently limited reduction rates. Our progress to date indicates that we are about half-way towards meeting that 15 percent goal. This goal builds on the progress made to date and expresses the Partnership's commitment to continue this important effort. We are continuing to look for opportunities to strengthen both the survey process and enforcement efforts to ensure that nursing homes are focused on non-pharmacologic approaches and residents are not receiving medications that do not have a clinical basis.

Ensuring Quality of Care by Putting Patients Over Paperwork

In addition to our monitoring and oversight of facilities, our Agency-wide efforts to return patients to the center of care by incentivizing improved quality and reducing provider burden play a critical, complementary role to our commitment to safeguarding the health of nursing home residents. Through our Patients Over Paperwork initiative[13], CMS is reducing provider burden and allowing clinicians to spend more

---

[12]https://www.cms.gov/newsroom/fact-sheets/data-show-national-partnership-improve-dementia-care-achieves- goals-reduce-unnecessary-antipsychotic

[13]https://www.cms.gov/Outreach-and-Education/Outreach/Partnerships/PatientsOverPaperwork.html

time with their patients – this is particularly important in a nursing home setting where residents have more complex care needs, and care decisions are often directed by family members. Reducing provider burden can also lower administrative costs, allowing facilities to dedicate their resources to other areas such as patient care.

CMS has been working tirelessly to evaluate and streamline regulations and operations with the goal to reduce unnecessary burden, increase efficiencies, and improve the customer experience. We have used several tactics to help us better understand burden related to nursing homes, from formal requests for information from stakeholders to engaging stakeholders directly to provide feedback to CMS on areas of burden. In a May 2017 proposed rule,[14] we stated that we are currently reviewing the nursing home requirements to balance the need to maintain quality of care while reducing procedural burdens on facilities. Specifically we noted that we are reviewing the requirements for obsolete or redundant provisions, areas where processes can be streamlined to reduce burden and cost, or other areas of possible elimination. We asked stakeholders for feedback in areas of burden placed by the revisions to the nursing home requirements and the potential impact of resident care and outcomes. We are considering potential changes to the requirements based on the feedback received.

In the Fiscal Year 2019 Skilled Nursing Facility Prospective Payment System Final Rule, CMS is moving towards a new patient-driven case-mix model system in Medicare to pay for services to residents in skilled nursing facilities. The new Patient-Driven Payment Model is designed to improve the incentives to treat the needs of the whole patient, instead of focusing on the volume of services the patient receives, which requires substantial paperwork to track over time. The Patient-Driven Payment Model simplifies complicated paperwork requirements for performing patient assessments by significantly reducing reporting burden (approximately $2.0 billion over 10 years), helping to create greater contact between health care professionals and their patients. This improved case-mix classification

---

[14] https://www.gpo.gov/fdsys/pkg/FR-2017-05-04/pdf/2017-08521.pdf

system moves Medicare towards a more value-based, unified post-acute care payment system that puts unique care needs of patients first while also significantly reducing administrative burden.

On September 7, 2017, CMS released a facility assessment tool[15] that helps a nursing home determine what resources are necessary to care for residents competently during both day-to-day operations and emergencies. The intent of the facility assessment is for the facility to evaluate its resident population and identify the resources needed to provide the necessary person-centered care and services the residents require. The tool may also be used by facilities to make decisions about direct care staff needs as well as capabilities to provide services to residents.

Promoting Transparency, Rewarding Quality, and Encouraging Competition

Skilled Nursing Facility Quality Reporting Program and Value-Based Purchasing Program

In recent years, we have undertaken a number of initiatives to promote higher quality and more efficient health care for Medicare beneficiaries. These initiatives include Skilled Nursing Facility Quality Reporting Program and Skilled Nursing Facility Value-Based Purchasing (VBP) Program. The overarching goal of these initiatives is to transform Medicare from a passive payer of claims to an active purchaser of quality health care for its beneficiaries.

The Skilled Nursing Facility Quality Reporting Program is authorized by the Social Security Act and applies to skilled nursing facilities and most swing-bed rural hospitals. The goal of the program is to use standardized quality measures and standardized data to enable interoperability and access to longitudinal information for providers to facilitate coordinated care, improved outcomes, and overall quality comparisons. Measures that are reported under the program include functional status, cognitive status, skin integrity, medication reconciliation, and major falls. In addition,

[15] https://qioprogram.org/facility-assessment-tool

measures on readmissions, discharge to community and Medicare spending per beneficiary are calculated using claims data, so skilled nursing facilities do not have to submit additional data for these measures. Under the program, skilled nursing facilities that fail to submit the required quality data to CMS are subject to a 2 percentage point reduction to the otherwise applicable annual market basket percentage update with respect to that fiscal year.

The implementation of the SNF VBP Program is an important step toward transforming how care is paid for, moving increasingly toward rewarding better value, outcomes, and innovations instead of merely volume. As required by law[16], beginning October 1, 2018, the SNF VBP Program will make positive or negative adjustments to the otherwise applicable payments under the Skilled Nursing Facility Prospective Payment System for services furnished by SNFs based on their performance on the program's readmissions measure. The single claims-based all cause 30-day hospital readmissions measure in the SNF VBP aims to improve individual outcomes through rewarding providers that take steps to limit the readmission of their patients to a hospital. Also as required by law, CMS will make available SNFs' performance under the SNF VBP Program, specifically including each SNF's performance score and the ranking of SNFs for each fiscal year.

Nursing Home Compare Five-Star Quality Rating System

Transparency is an important part of CMS's patient safety work and CMS is committed to making sure that patients and their families have the information they need to support their health care decisions for LTC facilities. CMS first created the Nursing Home Compare website in 1998 and has regularly increased the amount of information available to beneficiaries and their families about the quality of care in nursing homes participating in the Medicare and Medicaid programs.

CMS bases the five-star ratings of the Nursing Home Five Star Quality Rating System on an algorithm that calculates a composite view of nursing

---

[16] Section 1888(h) of the Social Security Act.

homes from three measures: results from their health inspections; performance on certain quality measures; and their staffing levels. CMS's Nursing Home Compare Website contains information for more than 15,000 Medicare and Medicaid nursing homes around the country. The website also includes detailed reports on facility health inspections, life safety code inspections and any identified noncompliance deficiency citations.

CMS has continually made improvements to Nursing Home Compare and the Five Star Quality Rating System to enhance and strengthen the comparison tool to provide the most accurate information to beneficiaries and their families. Throughout the years, CMS has added information to Nursing Home Compare, including information on facility ownership, federal administrative sanctions against nursing homes, and the full text of the nursing home health inspection reports. CMS implemented Nursing Home Compare 3.0 to strengthen and expand the Five Star Quality Rating System by adding quality measures, raising nursing home performance expectations, adjusting the methods for establishing staffing ratings, and expanding targeted surveys. In 2016, CMS expanded the number of quality measures included in Nursing Home Compare and the Five Star Quality Rating System. In April 2018, we replaced the data source for staffing information submitted by facilities through the Payroll-Based Journal system which improves the accuracy of the staffing information on Nursing Home Compare. CMS continues to work to improve Nursing Home Compare and the Five Star Quality Rating System. For example, in October 2018, we will be adding a measure of hospitalizations among long-stay residents as part of our continued efforts to improve quality and reduce costs.

Tracking Nursing Home Staffing Data

CMS has long identified staffing as one of the vital components of a nursing home's ability to provide quality care. Current law requires facilities to electronically submit direct care staffing information (including agency and contract staff) based on payroll and other auditable data. In 2015, CMS developed the Payroll-Based Journal system, which allows all facilities to submit their staffing data each quarter. The data, when combined with census information, is then used to calculate the level of staff in each nursing home. Last April, CMS began using the Payroll-Based Journal data to post staffing information on the Nursing Home Compare tool. This new staffing information is calculated using the number of hours facility staff are paid to work each day in a quarter, instead of the previous method of calculating staffing information using the total number of hours facility staff work over a two-week period. Also, unlike the previous data source, the new data are auditable back to payroll and other verifiable sources. These data provide unprecedented insight into how facilities are actually staffed, which can be used to analyze how facilities' staffing relates to quality and outcomes. In the future, we will also use this data to report on employee turnover and tenure, which also impacts the quality of care delivered.

While the new data warrants additional scrutiny and actions to ensure its accuracy and usefulness to consumers, we believe it will ultimately lead to improved staffing and result in better quality and care for nursing home residents. Already, the new data has helped us identify issues, such as significant variations in staffing between weekdays and weekends, and days with no registered nurse reported onsite. We are deeply concerned about these issues and are working with nursing homes to address them. For example, facilities who report seven or more days with no registered nurse hours are now assigned a one-star staffing quality rating. We are also planning to use the Payroll-Based Journal data to inform surveyors' investigations to help determine if staffing is an underlying cause of any quality issues. Furthermore, since the start of the program, we have been providing individualized feedback to each facility about their staffing data for them to use to improve the accuracy of future submissions. We will continue to accumulate and analyze the data to ensure that nursing homes are staffing their facilities appropriately in order to provide quality care to residents.

Moving Forward

Resident safety is our top priority in nursing homes that participate in the Medicare and Medicaid programs. We expect every nursing home to keep its residents safe and provide high quality care. CMS remains diligent in its duties to monitor nursing homes participating in Medicare and Medicaid across the country, and we look forward to continuing to work with Congress, states, facilities, residents and other stakeholders to make sure the residents we serve are receiving safe and high quality health care.

Mr. Harper. Thank you, Dr. Goodrich.

The chair will now recognize Ms. Dorrill for 5 minutes for the purposes of your opening statement.

STATEMENT OF RUTH ANN DORRILL

Ms. Dorrill. Good morning, Chairman Harper, Ranking Member DeGette, and other distinguished members of the subcommittee.

I have been visiting nursing homes on behalf of the OIG for 20 years. When you speak with the people who have chosen to spend their professional lives in these settings, they will tell you that nursing home care is incremental. By that I mean that the gains and the losses can be small and around the margins.

Nursing homes can be places of comfort and healing. They can make the difference between someone having 10 more good years or a downward spiral. But it's important to recognize that people who enter nursing homes are at low points at times of crisis. They often have not only an acute condition that landed them there in the first place, but they have many competing comorbidities and complex conditions on top of that.

Many of the facilities as you've said provide excellent care, but an alarming number of residents are subject to unsafe conditions, much of which is preventable with better guidance and government oversight. Our work has found widespread, serious problems in nursing home care and my remarks today will rest on three priority areas: harm to nursing home residents, emergency preparedness of nursing homes, and the important role of the state agencies.

First, in regard to harm, OIG has expended extensive time and focus on the problem of resident harm as it's been referenced already today, including harm from medical care known as adverse events. In a national study of hundreds of nursing homes, we found that a third of residents, 33 percent, one in three, were harmed by medical care—infections, blood clots, aspiration—and half of this harm, 59 percent, was preventable.

And an important point, one of the interesting things about this study to us was that most of these events weren't big, dramatic events that you think about when you think about harm or adverse events. Most of them were incremental. They were small. They were surrounding the daily, hourly care that's provided by certified nurse assistants and staffing throughout the nursing home.

And there are things that the staff didn't recognize and, in many cases, the family didn't recognize. The same is happening in hospitals. This low level, substandard care harms a tremendous number of people and we've recommended that CMS develop guidance and revise requirements for detecting and preventing this harm, the detection being a key component.

Residents also of course face abuse and neglect. In 2012, we found that only half of nursing homes were reporting allegations of abuse and neglect. And then we went back just last year in 2017 and looked at emergency room records and we found that it was still a substantial problem. There were many cases that were not reported by the nursing homes. We urged CMS at that time to take immediate action to monitor claims and to enforce against those who fail to report. OIG also works in the law enforcement side with our partners to hold accountable those who victimize residents.

Next, on emergency preparedness. So after Hurricane Katrina and other storms in 2005 we went into, we had found in looking at the deficiencies that almost all nursing homes met their emergency provisions. Ninety four percent were in compliance and yet when we visited a sample of homes who were actually affected by the hurricanes, we found that the plans weren't practical and up- to-date. That in many cases the nurses would pull out a pad and pen when they saw the hurricane coming as opposed to looking at the binder on the shelf.

We also found that once the storms hit and in their aftermath that whether the nursing homes evacuated or sheltered in place that they had problems with transportation, with staffing, with supplies, anything that you can imagine. We also found this for wildfires and for flooding.

When we went back, we also were struck by the fact that after additional storms—Ike, Gustav in 2009–2010—we found essentially the same thing, no improvement besides additional guidance by CMS. We recommended that CMS develop targeted guidance in requirements and as Dr. Goodrich said state agencies began assessing homes for these requirements last November.

Finally, I want to further emphasize the critical role of the state agencies in citing deficiencies when homes aren't up to snuff. In recent work, we found that seven of nine states did not consistently verify that homes actually corrected the deficiencies that the states had cited. In another study, we found that States weren't enforcing very critical core components, care and discharge planning, which are very important to patient outcomes. We recommended the States strengthen those procedures. And the report was in 2013, the recommendations were implemented just a few months ago in June of 2018.

In closing, the through line here is that while CMS has taken steps to create a framework for improvement, all progress will lie in the execution on the part of CMS, on the part of the state agencies, and on the part of the nursing homes. This means focused education and accountability from CMS and also staying alert to the impact of changes. Are the requirements understood, the new requirements by inspectors and homes are they practical? Do they improve care? None of that can really be assumed and the consequences are great.

OIG is recommending that CMS do more to protect nursing home residents and we are committed to that as well. We have ongoing work assessing a number of areas and we thank you for your ongoing leadership in this area and for the opportunity today.

[The prepared statement of Ms. Dorrill follows:]

U.S. DEPARTMENT OF HEALTH & HUMAN SERVICES
OFFICE OF INSPECTOR GENERAL

September 6, 2018

Good morning, Chairman Harper, Ranking Member DeGette, and other distinguished Members of the Subcommittee on Oversight and Investigations. Thank you for the opportunity to appear before you to discuss one of the most consequential issues in health care today: ensuring safe, quality care for residents in the Nation's nursing homes.

Key Takeaways

High-quality nursing homes can deliver enormous benefit as places of comfort and healing. For Medicare beneficiaries, nursing homes provide a clinically managed recovery period after illness and injury that can make the difference between more good years ahead or a downward spiral. For long-term-care residents and their families, often insured through Medicaid, nursing homes can provide responsible and much-needed care to those in fragile health.

Many nursing homes provide excellent care and are diligent in protecting their residents. But an alarming number of residents are subject to costly medical harm, unsafe conditions, and abuse and neglect, much of it preventable with better practices and oversight.

Nursing home care is a critical component of the continuum of care. Quality and safety of care in nursing homes affect the provision and cost of care in other settings. With an aging population and heightened focus on value-driven care, it is increasingly critical that Federal and State funds are used to purchase safe, high-quality care for vulnerable elderly and disabled patients.

Decades of OIG work on nursing homes has uncovered widespread problems in providing safe, high-quality care and reporting problems when they occur. We found that one in three Medicare residents in skilled nursing facilities experienced harm from the care provided, and half of these harm events were preventable. In addition, nursing homes affected by disasters, such as hurricanes, often struggle to execute emergency plans and protect residents. We have also raised concerns about failures to report potential cases of abuse and neglect. Criminal and civil enforcement actions have uncovered misconduct and grossly substandard care. State Agencies play a crucial role in ensuring quality and safety in nursing homes. However, OIG has found mixed results in these agencies' attention to nursing home deficiency corrections and complaints.

Addressing the challenge of improving nursing home safety and quality of care requires strong leadership by CMS and serious, sustained commitment and effort by CMS, States, and the provider community.

My testimony today will focus on significant OIG findings and recommendations regarding nursing home quality and safety in three key areas:

- Harm to residents in nursing homes
- Nursing home emergency preparedness
- State Agency enforcement

Overview of Accountability for Nursing Home Care and Oversight

According to CMS, Federal expenditures on nursing home care totaled $73 billion in 2016, including $44 billion for Medicaid long-term care and $29 billion for Medicare post-acute and other skilled care. Most nursing homes are certified to serve as both long-term-care facilities and skilled nursing facilities (SNFs). Long-term-care facilities provide health-related care and services needed as a result of a mental or physical condition and may serve beneficiaries whose condition may not rise to the level of needing skilled nursing care. SNFs provide skilled nursing care and rehabilitation services for residents who require such care because of injury, disability, or illness, typically following a hospital stay. Meeting the needs of these two different populations, long-term care and skilled post-acute care, can complicate the effective management of facilities, and make oversight more challenging.

CMS and States share responsibility for ensuring that nursing homes meet Federal requirements for quality and safety. State Agencies are required by CMS to conduct a "survey" (inspection) of nursing homes at least every 15 months to certify each facility's compliance. CMS oversees the State certification process and provides guidance regarding the survey process in its State Operations Manual (SOM) and Interpretive Guidelines.

When State Agencies identify deficiencies during their surveys, nursing homes must submit correction plans, and State Agencies must verify that the facility corrected its deficiencies. CMS and State Medicaid agencies may also take enforcement actions to address nursing home deficiencies, including imposing civil monetary penalties or terminating the nursing home from the Medicare Program, among other actions, as appropriate.

OIG Work Addressing harm to Residents in Nursing Homes

OIG Found that that One in Three SNF Residents Experienced Adverse Events during Their Nursing Home Stays, Including Infections, Pressure Ulcers, and Misuse of Medication

In a nation-wide review, OIG found that one-third of residents in SNFs experienced harm from the care provided in the nursing homes and more than half of the harm (adverse events) were preventable had the facilities provided better care. This report was one in a decade-long OIG series regarding adverse events in various healthcare settings, including hospitals.

The adverse events OIG identified in nursing homes resulted in a range of harmful outcomes for residents, including extended stays in the SNF, transfers to hospital emergency departments, and the need for life-sustaining intervention. For 6 percent of the adverse events, the harm contributed to residents' death. Over half of the residents who experienced harm returned to a hospital for treatment, incurring millions of dollars in additional Medicare expenditures.[17]

Some adverse events involved medical errors such as supplying incorrect medication, but most preventable harm resulted from daily substandard care, such as inadequate resident monitoring and failure or delay of necessary care. For these adverse events, residents and families may not know that they were harmed, thinking instead that the residents' suffering and decline were the result of their illness or conditions and inevitable. Nursing home staff also failed to identify harm in some cases; for example, a number of adverse events started with dehydration, which can quickly result in kidney damage. One nursing home resident died of cardiac arrest after progressive kidney failure that was not detected until the resident was awaiting discharge from the SNF.

Most nursing home residents who died or were harmed from adverse events had multiple, complex co-morbidities that made their care challenging. We found a wide range of adverse events not typically associated with nursing home care, such as internal bleeding due to medication. While some events are widely recognized as risks for patients in nursing homes, such as falls and pressure ulcers, fewer nursing home staff may be aware of the risks posed by aspiration and blood clots, both of which harmed numerous patients in our study sample. In our review of CMS and other guidance, we noted a tendency to focus narrowly on a subset of the most extreme harm events, many of which are rare, while missing the broad range of possible, more common harms that cause patient declines.

What is needed is a shift in thinking about the care provided in nursing homes. Our work identifying adverse events in nursing homes and other settings showed that nursing home residents often had care needs similar to patients in hospitals, with residents sometimes seriously ill and impaired. The hospital community has focused keenly on patient safety and, while still experiencing high harm rates in some categories, has made substantial

---

[17] OIG, *Adverse Events in Skilled Nursing Facilities: National Incidence Among Medicare Beneficiaries* (OEI-06-11-00370), issued February 2014. For this evaluation, OIG contracted with physicians who were experts in SNF care, surgery, cardiology, and infectious disease to conduct an extensive medical review of SNF stays.

changes in the provision of patient care and safety systems. Sustained improvements in nursing homes will require a cultural shift that recognizes clinical harm and elevates reduction of harm as a priority for nursing home care.

The foundation of OIG's recommendations to reduce harm is that CMS (and the Agency for Healthcare Research and Quality) raise awareness of adverse events in nursing homes (and other post-acute-care settings) with the same methods used to promote hospital safety. Broadening these and other patient safety improvement efforts to include the nursing home environment would ensure that safe care practices promoted in acute care hospitals extend to the critical periods of post-acute recovery and long-term care.

To address the high rate of harm in nursing homes, OIG made two recommendations to CMS: (1) provide guidance to nursing homes about detecting and reducing harm to be included in facility Quality Assurance and Performance Improvement programs, and (2) instruct State Agencies to review facility practices for identifying and reducing adverse events, and link related deficiencies specifically to resident safety practices. OIG determined that CMS fully implemented these recommendations on adverse events in SNFs as of August 2018. It is too early to assess the effectiveness of CMS's actions in changing practices, but they hold promise for improving quality of care and reducing adverse events for nursing home residents.

Meaningful improvement will rest on diligent execution by CMS and States, and continued evaluation of the effectiveness of these changes.

OIG has Raised Concerns about Failure to Report Allegations or potential Cases of Abuse and Neglect of Nursing Home Residents

It is both required and expected that nursing homes will report allegations of abuse or neglect to law enforcement or other appropriate agencies to ensure resident safety and protect victims of crimes. However, OIG has documented serious deficiencies in reporting of abuse and neglect of nursing home patients dating back several years and continuing in our recent and ongoing work. OIG found that, in 2012, nearly one in four nursing facilities did not have policies for reporting allegations of abuse or neglect and the subsequent results of an investigation, and facilities reported only half of allegations and investigation results as federally required.[18] In response to OIG recommendations that CMS ensure nursing homes maintain policies for reporting allegations of abuse or neglect and report allegations in a timely manner, CMS revised the SOM in 2017 to instruct State Agency surveyors to assess facility policies and practices.

Yet concerns about unreported abuse and neglect remain. OIG reviewed hospital emergency room records from 2015 and 2016 for SNF residents sent to hospitals whose injuries may have been the result of potential abuse or neglect in the SNF. In preliminary work, OIG found 134 such incidents across 33 States. We further found that many of these incidents may not have been reported to law enforcement. Pending completion of the full review, OIG alerted CMS that it had inadequate procedures to ensure that incidents of potential abuse and neglect at SNFs are properly identified and reported.[19] OIG made immediate suggestions for improvement, including that CMS analyze Medicare claims (including matching claims for emergency room services to claims for SNF services) to identify incidents of potential abuse and neglect and take specific steps to enhance its ability to impose civil monetary penalties for reporting failures.

OIG Investigations and Enforcement Cases Illustrate That Nursing Home Harm Can Involve Conduct by Individual Bad Actors, as Well Facility and Chain-Wide Conduct

OIG investigates potential criminal conduct and pursues enforcement actions to hold accountable those who victimize residents of nursing homes. In some cases, this involves criminal activity by bad actors. For example, in 2018, the owner of a long-term-care facility was convicted of

---

[18] OIG, *Nursing Facilities' Compliance with Federal Regulations for Reporting Allegations of Abuse or Neglect* (OEI-07-13-00010), issued in August 2014.

[19] OIG, *Early Alert: The Centers for Medicare & Medicaid Services Has Inadequate Procedures to Ensure That Incidents of Potential Abuse or Neglect at SNFs Are Identified and Reported in Accordance With Applicable Requirements* (A-01-17-00504), issued in August 2017.

engaging in the physical and emotional abuse of one of its residents, following an investigation by OIG and our law enforcement partners.

In other cases, facility-wide or chain-wide grossly substandard care can harm patients. Such cases may result in civil False Claims Act resolutions or administrative actions, such as exclusion. Patient neglect, often due to understaffing, is a recurring issue in False Claims Act cases. Other allegations that commonly arise in these cases include overmedication of nursing home residents, which may lead to falls and fractures; failure to follow physicians' orders; and failure to provide a habitable living environment, with concerns including mold and roof leaks.

Nursing Home Emergency Preparedness

Despite Enhanced Guidance from CMS, Nursing Homes Hit by Disaster Often Struggle to Execute Emergency Plans and Protect Residents

Nursing home residents and their families rely on facility administrators to plan and execute appropriate procedures during disasters. Through years of visiting nursing homes after disasters, we have learned that facilities may ostensibly meet CMS guidelines prior to the disaster, but at the time of crisis fail to follow requirements and prior planning.

In 2006, following Hurricanes Katrina, Rita, and others, OIG found that 94 percent of the Nation's nursing homes met Federal regulations for emergency plans. In visiting 20 nursing homes affected by hurricanes, however, we found that these plans were often not practical or up to date, and that during the crisis many administrators did not know how to navigate CMS guidelines and instructions from local authorities, and they often did not have adequate supplies, staffing, or transportation in place to care for residents. These findings indicated that State Agency reviews of emergency plans were insufficient, and that the plans themselves were often not useful.[20] In a followup study by OIG in 2012, after CMS had

---

[20] OIG, *Nursing Home Emergency Preparedness and Response during Recent Hurricanes* (OEI-06-06-00020), issued August 2006.

revised its guidance to include a suggested checklist for preparedness, we visited nursing homes affected by a range of disasters and found that only half had plans that included the checklist items.[21]

For nursing homes that continued to operate without adequate emergency planning, the omissions were often a matter of common sense and the consequences for residents extreme. One nursing home that flooded during a storm had no plan for responding to floods, despite residing in a flood plain. Other homes evacuated residents to facilities far away and without sufficient tracking or methods to ensure residents traveled with personal equipment and supplies, such as wheelchairs and medication. Administrators from most nursing homes that OIG studied reported that residents experienced deteriorating health conditions, skin issues, and falls resulting in serious injury. This occurred in nursing homes that evacuated and those that sheltered in place. In some cases of evacuation, residents' poor conditions necessitated hospitalization.

Reports of nursing homes' performance in the aftermath of the 2017 hurricanes—including failures to evacuate residents or to provide safe sheltering in place—raise continued questions about the adequacy of emergency plans and their proper execution.

OIG recommended that CMS require facilities to create effective emergency plans and take other specific actions in preparing for emergencies, such as improving staff training and communication with local authorities. In 2016, CMS revised its emergency preparedness requirements for nursing homes and other healthcare facilities that participate in Medicare and Medicaid, to include specific provisions for planning, training, and communication. State Agencies began assessing compliance for these provisions in November 2017. OIG will continue to monitor these important provisions.

---

[21] OIG, *Gaps Continue To Exist in Nursing Home Preparedness and Response After Disasters* (OEI-06-09-00270), issued April 2012.

State Agency Enforcement

State Agencies Play a Critical Role in Ensuring the Quality and Safety of Nursing Homes, and OIG has Found Mixed Results in State Agency Attention to Nursing Home Deficiencies

From 2015 to 2018, OIG completed audits of nine States to determine whether the State Agency took appropriate steps to verify that nursing facilities had corrected identified deficiencies. OIG found that State Agencies in seven of nine States were not meeting requirements to verify correction of deficiencies.[22] Lack of verification was evident in both serious and minor deficiencies. For example, surveyors found that a nursing home failed to provide a resident oxygen per physician orders; the corrective action plan included additional training for nursing staff. Yet the State Agency was unable to confirm that the staff involved attended the training.

OIG also found that one of the nine States reviewed did not conduct standard surveys for approximately 40 percent of nursing homes within the required 15 months. For seven States that did not meet requirements, OIG recommended that State Agencies improve verification processes, update internal systems, and for the one State, develop a correction plan to ensure the State conducts timely surveys. OIG found that the remaining two States were in full compliance. Four of the States with recommendations implemented them, including the State not performing timely surveys. Recommendations for three of the States remain outstanding, including two States that received our audit reports only within the last few months.

Other OIG findings indicated that State Agency oversight of SNFs was not sufficient to ensure that SNFs developed and followed care and discharge plans for residents, as required. These care and discharge plans can be the linchpin of effective SNF care, helping to ensure that residents receive needed care, protecting residents from receiving unnecessary care,

---

[22] OIG's State audits included Arizona (A-09-16-02013), Florida (A-04-17-08052), Kansas (A-07-1703218), Missouri (A-07-16-03217), Nebraska (A-07-17-03224), New York (A-02-15-01024), North Carolina (A-04-17-02500), Oregon (A-09-16-02007), and Washington (A-09-13-02039).

and assisting them in securing home- and community-based care and personal care services that can prevent them from re-entering the SNF or a hospital.

OIG made extensive recommendations to CMS that the agency address this problem from multiple vantage points: (1) strengthen the regulations on care and discharge planning, (2) provide guidance to SNFs to improve planning, (3) increase surveyor efforts to identify problems, (4) link payments to meeting quality-of-care requirements, and (5) follow up on the SNFs that failed to meet requirements.[23] In June 2018, OIG determined that CMS had fully implemented these recommendations. We will continue to monitor the extent to which CMS's and State Agencies' actions resolve the problems and improve care.

State Agencies serve as front-line responders to address health and safety complaints in nursing homes. State Agencies are responsible for onsite investigations of serious complaints of abuse and neglect. OIG work in 2017 found that a few states fell short in timely investigations of the two most serious categories of complaints: immediate jeopardy and high priority.[24]

Next Steps to Improve Nursing Home Quality and Safety

Sustained Commitment by CMS and Continued Collaboration among HHS, States, Providers, and Residents and Their Families will be Critical to Ensuring Quality and Safety

Quality nursing home care requires a partnership between a large and diverse group of Federal, State, and local entities. Residents and their families are also critical stakeholders. As the Federal agency charged with oversight of nursing home compliance and performance, CMS must demonstrate strong leadership of this group. Effective collaboration will narrow gaps, provide better information and insight, and give greater

---

[23] OIG, *Skilled Nursing Facilities Often Fail to Meet Care Planning and Discharge Requirements* (OEI-02-09-00201), issued February 2013.

[24] OIG, *A Few States Fell Short in Timely Investigations of the Most Serious Nursing Home Complaints: 2011-2015* (OEI-01-16-00330), issued September 2017.

assurance to residents and their families that they will receive high-quality care.

As an example, following the 2011 OIG report *Medicare Atypical Antipsychotic Drug Claims for Elderly Nursing Home Residents*, CMS led an effort across HHS to correct improper drug prescribing and use in nursing homes. OIG found that 83 percent of atypical antipsychotic drug claims were for elderly nursing home residents not diagnosed with a condition for which the Food and Drug Administration (FDA) had approved antipsychotic medications. This supported a theory long held by residents' advocates that nursing homes used atypical antipsychotic medications for "off-label" indications, with the purpose of controlling undesirable behavior. Both CMS and FDA took action to make changes to regulations and guidance, and CMS formed a public-private effort, the National Partnership to Improve Dementia Care in Nursing Homes, to engage providers, advocates, and families. Subsequent CMS data show substantial reductions in the use of these drugs among nursing home residents. Given the number of stakeholders involved and the urgency of the problems, this type of public-private partnership would be useful for CMS to foster improvements across nursing home care.

Further, it is critical that States remain active participants in the Federal-State partnership needed to oversee nursing homes. States are on the front line in surveying nursing homes, identifying deficiencies, and verifying corrections. States play an essential enforcement role when residents are victims of abuse and neglect. States' active participation in ensuring that nursing homes are providing safe, high-quality care is essential to improving patient outcomes and reducing adverse events.

To Protect Nursing Home Residents, OIG Will Continue to Assess CMS Oversight and Nursing Home and State Agency Performance, Monitor the Impact of Program Changes, and Use our Enforcement Tools to Address Misconduct

Nursing home residents deserve and should expect high-quality care and to be safe from abuse and neglect. OIG will continue to monitor whether CMS's recent actions to improve safety and quality produce the intended positive outcomes. Moreover, OIG will follow up on its findings and recommendations to State Agencies to strengthen the effectiveness of their efforts.

OIG has upcoming work that will assess multiple dimensions of nursing home quality and safety to protect beneficiaries. These audits and evaluations follow up on past findings and recommendations, and examine new areas, such as nursing home compliance with new Life and Safety Code requirements, assessment of the accuracy and use of new nursing home staffing data, and the extent to which State Agencies investigate involuntary resident transfers and discharges.

Allegations involving patient harm remain a top OIG enforcement priority. OIG will continue to investigate potential criminal conduct and pursue administrative actions to hold accountable those who victimize residents of nursing homes. In resolving False Claims Act cases, OIG may enter into "quality of care" corporate integrity agreements (CIAs) with nursing homes or chains that require actions to improve quality of care and safety. OIG is currently monitoring quality of care CIAs covering more than 200 nursing homes. OIG also collaborates closely with the 50 State Medicaid Fraud Control Units (MFCUs) that often have primary responsibility for enforcement of cases of abuse and neglect in nursing homes.

Call to Action

To provide guidance, support, and oversight of this industry is a grave and vitally important responsibility. Government policies and leadership, Federal and State, can substantially affect residents' experience and outcomes. The problems I present today are not new, and they may seem daunting and intractable given the challenges and complexities of nursing home care. But change is possible, and essential. Nursing home care will always be a deeply challenging enterprise, but with dedicated attention and focus, CMS, States, and providers can do better.

While CMS has taken steps to create a framework for correcting problems of resident harm and risk, all progress will be in the execution of that framework and the performance of CMS, States, and providers. CMS must stay alert to the impact of policies and practices and promote meaningful, sustainable change. OIG is committed to working with CMS as it takes action to address problems identified by our work, the Government Accountability Office, and others.

Thank you for your ongoing leadership in this area and for affording OIG the opportunity to testify and discuss with you this vitally important topic.

Mr. Harper. Thank you, Ms. Dorrill.

We will now recognize Mr. Dicken for 5 minutes for the purposes of his opening statement. Thank you.

STATEMENT OF JOHN DICKEN

Mr. Dicken. Chairman Harper, Ranking Member DeGette, and members of the subcommittee, I'm pleased to be here today to discuss GAO's body of work on nursing home quality and the Center for Medicaid and Medicaid Services oversight of nursing homes.

For many years, GAO has reported on problems in nursing home quality and weaknesses in CMS' oversight. As early as 1998, GAO reported that despite Federal and State oversight, certain California nursing homes were not sufficiently monitored to guarantee the safety and welfare of their residents. In the intervening 2 decades across more than two dozen reports, GAO has consistently found shortcomings in the care that some nursing home residents received and in Federal and State oversight of nursing homes.

In response to identified weaknesses, CMS and state survey agencies have made a number of changes in their oversight. Inspection protocols have been updated, enforcement tools have been revised, and consumers have been provided more information to compare nursing homes. Yet, we continue to see mixed results in indicators intended to assess the quality of care. Further, we lack full assurance of these indicators including information made available to consumers are consistently based on accurate data and we remain concerned that the prevalence of serious care problems remains unacceptably high.

In my remaining time I'd like to briefly summarize key takeaways from GAO reports issued in 2015 and 2016 that examine trends in nursing home quality, information made available to consumers for comparing nursing homes, and changes CMS had made to its oversight activities. I will also note CMS' responses to recommendations we made.

First, we found that data on nursing home quality showed mixed results. We found an increase in reported consumer complaints through 2014, suggesting that consumers' concerns about nursing home quality increased. In contrast, trends in care deficiencies, nurse staffing levels, and clinical quality indicators through 2014 indicate potential improvement.

Second, we found data issues complicated the ability to assess quality trends. For example, at that time CMS allowed states to use different survey methodologies to measure deficiencies in nursing home care. GAO recommended CMS implement a standardized survey methodology across states and in November 2017 CMS completed national implementation. Further, GAO recommended CMS implement a plan for ongoing auditing of quality data that had been self-reported by nursing homes. The agency concurred and has begun auditing staffing data that now relies on payroll-based reporting, but CMS does not have a plan to audit certain other quality data on a continuing basis.

Third, in the 2016 report we found CMS did not systematically prioritize recommended changes to improve its Nursing Home Compare website. In several factors it limited consumers' ability to use CMS' five-star rating system. CMS agreed with these recommendations and earlier this year completed actions establishing a process to prioritize website improvements and adding explanatory information about the five-star system. But CMS has not yet acted on other recommendations including providing national comparison information that could help consumers better make distinctions between nursing homes.

Fourth, CMS had modified certain oversight activities at the time of our 2015 report and those steps have continued. Some modifications expanded activities such as creating new training for state surveys on unnecessary medication use, others reduced existing activities. For example, CMS reduced the scope of Federal monitoring surveys which may decrease CMS' ability to monitor whether state survey agencies understate serious care deficiencies. Similarly, CMS reduced the number of homes designated as special focus facilities which may limit its ability to monitor homes with poor performance. GAO recommended CMS monitor the effects of these modifications and CMS indicates it is beginning to take steps to do so.

In closing, addressing the long-term concerns that nursing residents receive unacceptable care requires sustained Federal and state commitment. We maintain the importance of monitoring to help CMS better understand how oversight modifications affect nursing home quality and to improve its oversight given limited resources.

Chairman Harper, Ranking Member DeGette, and members of the subcommittee, this concludes my prepared statement. I'd be pleased to answer any questions that you may have.

[The prepared statement of Mr. Dicken follows:]

NURSING HOME QUALITY: CONTINUED IMPROVEMENTS NEEDED IN CMS'S DATA AND OVERSIGHT

Why GAO Did This Study

Approximately 15,600 nursing homes participating in the Medicare and Medicaid programs provide care to 1.4 million residents—a population of elderly and disabled individuals. To help ensure nursing home residents receive quality care, CMS defines quality standards that homes must meet to participate in the Medicare and Medicaid programs. To monitor compliance with these standards, CMS enters into agreements with state survey agencies to conduct on-site surveys of the state's homes and also collects other data on nursing home quality.

Although CMS and others have reported some potential improvements in nursing home quality, questions have been raised about nursing home quality and weaknesses in CMS oversight.

This statement summarizes GAO's October 2015 report, GAO-16-33. Specifically, it describes (1) trends in nursing home quality through 2014, and (2) changes CMS had made to its oversight activities as of October 2015. It also includes the status of GAO's recommendations associated with these findings. GAO recently obtained information from CMS officials about steps they have taken to implement the 2015 GAO recommendations.

What GAO Found

GAO's October 2015 report found mixed results in nursing home quality based on its analysis of trends reflected in key sources of quality data that the Centers for Medicare & Medicaid Services (CMS) collects.

- An increase in reported consumer complaints suggested that consumers' concerns about nursing home quality increased.
- In contrast, trends in care deficiencies, nurse staffing levels, and clinical quality measures indicated potential improvement in nursing home quality.

GAO also found that data issues complicated CMS's ability to assess nursing home quality trends. For example:

- CMS allowed states to use different survey methodologies to measure deficiencies in nursing home care, which complicates the ability to make comparisons nationwide. GAO recommended that CMS implement a standardized survey methodology across states, and in November 2017 CMS completed national implementation.

- CMS did not regularly audit selected quality data including nurse staffing and clinical data (for example, on residents with pressure ulcers) to ensure their accuracy. GAO recommended CMS implement a plan for ongoing auditing of quality data. The agency concurred with this recommendation and has been conducting regular audits of nurse staffing data but does not have a plan to audit other quality data on a continuing basis. GAO continues to believe that regular audits are needed to ensure the accuracy and comparability of nursing home quality data.

GAO's October 2015 report found that CMS had made numerous modifications to its nursing home oversight activities. However, CMS had not monitored how the modifications might affect its ability to assess nursing home quality. GAO found that some modifications expanded or added new activities—such as creating new training for state surveyors on unnecessary medication usage— while others reduced existing activities. For example, CMS reduced the number of nursing homes participating in the Special Focus Facility program—which provides additional oversight of certain homes with a history of poor performance—by over half from 2013 to 2014. CMS officials told GAO that some of the reductions to oversight activities were in response to an increase in oversight responsibilities and a limited number of staff and financial resources. To help ensure modifications do not adversely affect CMS's ability to assess nursing home quality, GAO recommended that CMS monitor modifications of essential oversight activities to better understand the effects on nursing home quality oversight. CMS concurred with this recommendation and told us it has begun to take steps to address it. Such monitoring is important for CMS to better understand how its oversight modifications affect nursing home quality and to improve its oversight given limited resources.

Chairman Harper, Ranking Member DeGette, and Members of the Subcommittee:

I'm pleased to be here today to discuss our work on nursing home quality and the Centers for Medicare & Medicaid Services' (CMS) oversight of nursing homes. Nationwide, approximately 15,600 nursing homes provide care to about 1.4 million nursing home residents—a population of elderly and disabled individuals. To help ensure this population receives quality care, CMS defines the quality standards nursing homes must meet in order to participate in the Medicare and Medicaid programs.[25] To monitor compliance with these standards, CMS enters into agreements with state survey agencies to conduct required surveys, or evaluations, of the state's nursing homes.

For many years, we and the Department of Health and Human Services (HHS) Office of the Inspector General (OIG) have reported on problems in nursing home quality and on weaknesses in CMS's oversight.[26] As early as 1998, GAO reported on residents in California nursing homes who received unacceptable care that sometimes endangered their health and safety.[27] In the intervening two decades, across more than 20 reports, GAO has repeatedly reported on shortcomings both in the care some nursing home residents received and in the federal and state oversight of nursing home care. For example, a 1999 report found that complaint investigation processes were often inadequate to protect residents, and a 2008 report found federal oversight continued to demonstrate that state inspections understated serious care problems.[28] In response to identified weaknesses, CMS and state survey agencies have made some changes in how they conduct oversight of nursing home quality, and some potential improvements in nursing home quality have been reported in recent years. For example, CMS has reported a decrease in the percentage of homes that

---

[25] Medicaid, a federal-state health financing program for low-income and medically needy individuals, is the nation's primary payer of long-term services and supports for children and adults with disabilities and aged individuals. Medicare, the federal health insurance program for people age 65 and older, individuals under age 65 with certain disabilities, and individuals diagnosed with end-stage renal disease, covers some short-term skilled nursing and rehabilitative care for beneficiaries following an acute care hospital stay.

[26] See, for example, OIG, *Adverse Events in Skilled Nursing Facilities: National Incidence Among Medicare Beneficiaries*, OEI-06-11-00370 (Washington, D.C.: Feb. 2014).

[27] See GAO, *California Nursing Homes: Care Problems Persist Despite Federal and State Oversight*, GAO/HEHS-98-202 (Washington, D.C.: July 27, 1998).

[28] See GAO, *Nursing Homes: Complaint Investigation Processes Often Inadequate to Protect Residents,* HEHS-99-80 (Washington, D.C.: Mar. 22, 1999 and *Nursing Homes: Federal Monitoring Surveys Demonstrate Continued Understatement of Serious Care Problems and CMS Oversight Weaknesses*, GAO-08-517 (Washington, D.C.: May 9, 2008).

were cited for serious health deficiencies from 2006 to 2014.[29] In addition, CMS and others have reported on improvements in specific nursing home clinical measures, such as reductions in the use of physical restraints, which can be a sign of improved quality of care.

However, as you know, news stories and reports continue to identify potential problems in nursing homes. For example, a July 2018 article from *Kaiser Health News* highlighted that new data collected by CMS to evaluate nurse staffing showed most nursing homes had fewer nurses and caretaking staff than they had previously reported to CMS, with frequent and significant fluctuations in day-to-day staffing.[30] As part of its ongoing work, the OIG determined CMS does not have adequate procedures in place to ensure incidents of potential abuse or neglect of Medicare beneficiaries in nursing homes are identified and reported.[31] In light of these concerns and a delay in enforcement of 2016 long-term care regulatory reforms, as well as a reduction in civil money penalties for non-compliance with federal health and safety requirements, 17 state attorneys general sent a letter urging CMS to implement the strengthened regulations and maintain penalties for non-compliance in May 2018.[32]

To help inform today's discussion, my testimony will focus on the findings from our October 2015 report examining CMS's oversight of nursing home quality.[33] In particular, this statement will address:

---

[29] CMS, *Nursing Home Data Compendium 2015 Edition.*

[30] J. Rau, "Like a Ghost Town: Erratic Nursing Home Staffing Revealed Through New Records." *Kaiser Health News*, July 13, 2018, accessed August 27, 2018. https:// khn.org/news/like-a-ghost-town-erratic-nursing-home-staffing-revealed-through- new-records/

[31] See Daniel R. Levinson, OIG, HHS, memorandum to Seema Verma, Administrator, CMS, *Early Alert: The Centers for Medicare & Medicaid Services Has Inadequate Procedures To Ensure That Incidents of Potential Abuse or Neglect at Skilled Nursing Facilities Are Identified and Reported in Accordance With Applicable Requirements*, A-01-17-00504 (Aug. 24, 2017).

[32] Attorneys General of California, Connecticut, the District of Columbia, Hawaii, Illinois, Iowa, Maryland, Massachusetts, Minnesota, Mississippi, New York, Oregon, Pennsylvania, Rhode Island, Vermont, Virginia, and Washington, letter to the Secretary of Health and Human Services and Administrator of CMS, *Regulation of Skilled Nursing Facilities* (May 30, 2018).

[33] See GAO, *Nursing Home Quality: CMS Should Continue to Improve Data And Oversight*, GAO-16-33 (Washington, D.C.: Oct. 30, 2015).

1. trends in nursing home quality through 2014, and
2. changes CMS had made to its oversight activities as of October 2015.

In addition, I will highlight key actions that we recommended HHS take, including HHS's response and the current status of those recommendations.

While my comments today focus on the findings of our October 2015 report, they are also informed by our large body of work examining nursing home quality. (See Appendix I for a list of related GAO reports.)

In our October 2015 report, we analyzed four key sets of quality data from CMS using the most recent data available at that time. We also reviewed relevant oversight and data documents and interviewed officials from CMS central office, CMS regional offices, and state survey agencies for a selected group of states. The 2015 report includes a full description of our scope and methodology. We also obtained information from CMS on the status of our 2015 recommendations, as of 2018. We conducted the work on which this statement is based in accordance with generally accepted government auditing standards. Those standards require that we plan and perform the audit to obtain sufficient, appropriate evidence to provide a reasonable basis for our findings and conclusions based on our audit objectives. We believe that the evidence obtained provides a reasonable basis for our findings and conclusions based on our audit objectives.

Background

Oversight of nursing homes is a shared federal-state responsibility, with CMS central and regional offices overseeing activities completed by state survey agencies.

Specifically, CMS central office (1) oversees the federal quality standards nursing homes must meet to participate in the Medicare and Medicaid programs and (2) establishes the responsibilities of CMS's regional offices and state survey agencies to ensure federal quality standards for nursing homes are met. CMS regional offices oversee state activities and report results back to CMS central office. Specifically, regional offices are required to conduct annual federal monitoring surveys to assess the adequacy of surveys conducted by state survey agencies. CMS regional offices also evaluate state surveyors' performance on factors such as the frequency and quality of state surveys. Finally, in each state, under agreement with CMS, a state survey agency assesses whether nursing homes meet CMS's standards by conducting regular surveys and investigations of complaints regarding resident care or safety, as needed.

CMS collects data on nursing home quality through annual standard surveys and complaint investigations, as well as other sources, such as staffing data and clinical quality measures.

- Standard surveys. By law, every nursing home receiving Medicare or Medicaid payment must undergo a standard survey during which teams of state surveyors conduct a comprehensive on-site evaluation of compliance with federal quality standards.[34] Nursing homes with consistently poor performance can be selected for the Special Focus Facility (SFF) program, which requires more intensive oversight, including more frequent surveys.[35]

---

[34] For most deficiencies identified during surveys, a home is required to prepare a plan of correction, and, depending on the severity of the deficiency, surveyors may conduct a revisit to ensure that the nursing home has implemented its plan and corrected the deficiency. The scope and severity of a deficiency determine the enforcement actions— such as requiring training for staff, imposing monetary penalties, or termination from the Medicare and Medicaid programs.

[35] According to CMS guidance, SFF nursing homes that fail to significantly improve after three standard surveys, or about 18 months, may be involuntarily terminated from Medicare and Medicaid. The SFF program is statutorily required, and CMS is mandated to conduct its SFF program for homes that have "substantially failed" to meet applicable requirements of the Social Security Act. For more information on the SFF program, see GAO, *Poorly Performing Nursing Homes: Special Focus Facilities Are Often Improving, but CMS's Program Could Be Strengthened*, GAO-10-197 (Washington, D.C.: Mar. 19, 2010).

- Complaint investigations. Nursing homes also are surveyed on an as-needed basis with investigations of consumer complaints. These complaints can be filed with state survey agencies by residents, families, ombudsmen, or others acting on a resident's behalf. During an investigation, state surveyors evaluate the nursing home's compliance with a specific federal quality standard.
- Staffing data. Nurse staffing levels are considered a key component of nursing home quality and are often measured in total nurse hours per resident day. Higher nurse staffing levels are typically linked with higher quality nursing home care.
- Clinical quality measures. Nursing homes are required to provide data on certain clinical quality measures—such as the incidence of pressure ulcers—for all residents to CMS. CMS currently tracks data for 18 clinical quality measures.

CMS publicly reports a summary of each nursing home's quality data on its Nursing Home Compare website using a five-star quality rating.[36] The Five-Star Quality Rating System assigns each nursing home an overall rating and three component ratings—surveys (standard and complaint), staffing, and quality measures—based on the extent to which the nursing home meets CMS's quality standards and other measures. In a 2016 report, we found that CMS did not have a systematic process for prioritizing recommended changes to improve its Nursing Home Compare website and that several factors limited the ability of CMS's Five-Star Quality Rating System to help consumers understand nursing home quality and choose a home. We recommended that CMS establish a process to evaluate and prioritize website improvements and add explanatory information about the Five-Star System to Nursing Home Compare.

---

[36] See GAO, *Nursing Homes: Consumers Could Benefit from Improvements to the Nursing Home Compare Website and Five-Star Quality Rating System*, GAO-17-61 (Washington, D.C.: Nov. 18, 2016) and *Health Care Transparency: Actions Needed to Improve Cost and Quality Information for Consumers*, GAO-15-11 (Washington, D.C.: Oct. 20, 2014).

HHS agreed and in 2018 completed actions on these recommendations, but has not yet acted on the other recommendations, including providing national comparison information that we maintain are important to help enable consumers to understand nursing home quality and make distinctions between nursing homes.

Nursing Home Quality Data Show Mixed Results, Although Data Issues Complicate Ability to Assess Quality Trends

In our October 2015 report examining trend data that give insight into nursing home quality, we found that four key data sets showed mixed results, and data issues complicated the ability to assess quality trends.

Data on Nursing Home Quality Showed Mixed Results

Nationally, one of the four data sets—consumer complaints—suggested consumers' concerns over nursing home quality increased from 2005 to 2014. However, the other three data sets—deficiencies, staffing levels, and clinical quality measures—indicated potential improvement in nursing home quality (see Table 1). Specifically, we found consumer complaints—which can originate from residents, families, ombudsmen, or others acting on a resident's behalf—had a 21 percent increase from 2005 to 2014. In contrast, nurse staffing levels increased 9 percent from 2009 to 2014 and selected quality measure scores showed decreases in the number of reported quality problems, such as falls resulting in major injury from 2011 to 2014.

In addition, we identified 416 homes in 36 states that had consistently poor performance across the four data sets we examined. Of the 416 homes, 71 (17 percent) were included in the Special Focus Facility (SFF) program at some point between 2005 and 2014.

Table 1. Overview of Trends in Key Nursing Home Quality Data

Quality data	Description	Time period	Change[a]
Consumer complaints	Average number of consumer complaints reported per nursing home	2005-2014	Increase in complaints (21%)
Deficiencies cited on standard surveys	Average number of serious deficiencies—deficiencies that, at a minimum, caused harm to the resident cited per nursing home surveyed	2005-2014	Decrease in serious deficiencies (41%)
Nurse staffing	Average total nurse hours per resident day[b]	2009-2014	Increase in nurse hours (9%)
Selected quality measures	Nursing homes' scores on 8 of CMS's clinical nursing home quality measures[c]	2011-2014	Decrease in quality problems (varied by measure)

Source: GAO analysis of Centers for Medicare & Medicaid Services (CMS) data. | GAO-18-694T

[a] Specifically, from 2005 through 2014, the average number of consumer complaints reported per nursing home increased nationally from 3.2 to 3.9. From 2005 through 2014, the number of serious deficiencies cited per nursing home surveyed decreased nationally from 0.35 to 0.21. From 2009 through 2014, the average total nurse hours per resident per day increased nationally from 4.2 to 4.6. From 2011 through 2014, nationwide nursing homes' scores on all 8 of our selected quality measures improved, at least somewhat, but the rate of decline varied greatly by quality measure. For example, the percentage of long-stay residents with too much weight loss decreased 1.3 percent over the 4-year period, while the percentage of short-stay residents with new or worsening pressure ulcers decreased 52.2 percent.

[b] The average total nurse hours per resident per day is a measure of registered nurse, licensed practical nurse, and nurse assistant hours. At the time of our 2015 report this measure was based on the number of hours worked that nursing homes self-reported; as of July 2016, these measures were based on payroll and other verifiable data submitted to CMS by the homes.

[c] The selected quality measures include the percentage of long-stay residents who report moderate to severe pain; the percentage of long-stay, high-risk residents with pressure ulcers; the percentage of long-stay residents who lose too much weight; the percentage of long-stay residents who were physically restrained; the percentage of long-stay residents experiencing one or more falls with major injury; the percentage of long-stay residents who received antipsychotic medication; the percentage of short-stay residents who report moderate to severe pain; and the percentage of short-stay residents with pressure ulcers that are new or worsening.

Data Issues Complicated CMS's Ability to Assess Quality Trends

In our October 2015 report, we found CMS's ability to use available data to assess nursing home quality trends was complicated by various issues with these data, which made it difficult to determine whether observed trends reflect actual changes in quality, data issues, or both. CMS has taken some actions to address these data complications, however, more work is needed.

Consumer Complaints

The average number of consumer complaints reported per nursing home increased in the 10 years of data we examined, although it is unclear to what extent this can be attributed to a change in quality or to state variation in the recording of complaints. Some state survey agency officials explained that changes in how they recorded complaints into CMS's complaint tracking system could in part account for the jump in reported complaints. In addition, officials at one state survey agency explained the increase in complaints could also reflect state-level efforts to provide consumers with more user-friendly options for filing complaints. Similarly, in April 2011, we found differences in how states record and track complaints.[37]

Deficiencies cited on Standard Surveys

The decline in the number of serious deficiencies—deficiencies that at a minimum caused a harm to the resident—in the data we examined may have indicated an improvement in quality, although it may also be attributed to inconsistencies in measurement. For example, the use of multiple survey types, such as both traditional paper-based surveys and electronic surveys, to conduct the standard survey that every nursing home receiving Medicare or Medicaid payment must undergo complicates the ability to compare the results of these surveys nationally.[38] In our October 2015 report, we recommended CMS implement the same survey methodology across all states; HHS agreed with this recommendation and in November 2017 completed its national implementation of this electronic survey methodology.[39]

---

[37] See GAO, *Nursing Homes: More Reliable Data and Consistent Guidance Would Improve CMS Oversight of State Complaint Investigations*, GAO-11-280 (Washington, D.C.: Apr. 7, 2011).

[38] Some regional offices and state survey agencies we spoke to for the October 2015 report noted electronic surveys result in fewer deficiencies cited, especially for more serious deficiencies and deficiencies related to quality of care. Thus, the decreasing trend of serious deficiencies could be the result of an expanding use of electronic surveys, rather than an improvement in the quality of nursing homes.

[39] CMS, letter to State Survey Agency Directors, *Revision to State Operations Manual (SOM) Appendix PP for Phase 2, F-Tag Revisions, and Related Issues*, S&C: 17-36-NH (June 30, 2017).

Nurse Staffing

CMS data showed the average total nurse hours per resident day increased from 2009 through 2014, although CMS did not have assurance these data were accurate. Many of the regional office and state survey agency officials we spoke with expressed concern over the self-reported nature of these data, noting that it may be easy to misrepresent nurse staff hours. At the time of our 2015 report, CMS was in the process of implementing a system to collect staffing information based on payroll and other verifiable data and has now completed that implementation, as required by law. We recommended in 2015 that CMS establish and implement a clear plan for ongoing auditing of its staffing data and other quality data. HHS agreed with this recommendation and in July 2018 CMS provided us with documentation that it was conducting regular audits of this new nurse staffing data. According to CMS, facilities experienced challenges submitting complete and accurate data in the early stages, however, as of April 2018 the agency has begun relying on the payroll data to calculate the staffing measures that it posts in Nursing Home Compare and uses in the Five-Star Quality Rating System.[40]

Selected Quality Measures

Nursing homes generally improved their performance on the eight selected quality measures we reviewed, although it is unclear to what extent this can be attributed to a change in quality or possible inaccuracies in self-reported data. Like the nurse staffing data used by CMS, data on nursing homes' performance on these measures were self-reported, and until 2014 CMS conducted little to no auditing of these data to ensure their accuracy. In our 2015 report, we found CMS had begun taking steps to help mitigate the problem with self- reported data by starting to audit the data in 2015; however, the agency did not have clear plans to continue the audits beyond 2016. As such, in our recommendation we indicated the need for ongoing auditing of data used to calculate clinical quality measures. As of August 2018, CMS has not provided us a plan for ongoing

[40] See CMS, letter to State Survey Agency Directors, *Transition to Payroll-Based Journal (PBJ) Staffing Measures on the Nursing Home Compare Tool on Medicare.gov and the Five Star Quality Rating System* (April 6, 2018, QSO-18-17-NH).

auditing of its clinical quality measures and we continue to believe that CMS should establish and carry out such a plan.

Collectively, these data issues have broader implications related to nursing home quality trends, including potential effects on the quality benchmarks CMS sets and consumers' decisions about which nursing home to select.[41] Furthermore, data used by CMS to assess quality measures are also used when determining Medicare payments to nursing homes, so data issues—and CMS's internal controls related to the data—could affect the accuracy of payments. Moreover, the use of quality data for payment purposes will expand in fiscal year 2019 when a nursing home value-based purchasing program will be implemented, which will increase or reduce Medicare payments to nursing homes based on certain quality measures.

CMS had Modified Oversight Activities by 2015, but had not Monitored Potential Effect on Nursing Home Quality Oversight

Our 2015 report found that CMS had made numerous modifications to its nursing home oversight activities in recent years, but had not monitored the potential effect of these modifications on nursing home quality oversight. Some of these modifications expanded or added new oversight activities—for example, CMS expanded the number of tools available to state surveyors when investigating medication-related adverse events, increased the amount of nursing home quality data available to the public, and created new trainings for surveyors on unnecessary medication usage.[42] However, other modifications reduced existing oversight activities.

In 2015, we highlighted modifications that reduced two existing oversight activities—the federal monitoring survey program and the SFF program.

---

[41] In our 2016 report on CMS's Nursing Home Compare and Five-Star Quality Rating System, we reviewed the extent to which the rating system—which is based on these data sets—enables consumers to understand nursing home quality and make distinctions between homes. See GAO-17-61.

[42] See GAO-16-33 for additional information on oversight modifications made.

- Federal monitoring surveys: CMS reduced the scope of the federal monitoring surveys regional offices use to evaluate state surveyors' skills in assessing nursing home quality. CMS requires regional offices to complete federal monitoring surveys in at least 5 percent of nursing homes surveyed by the state each year. Starting in 2013, CMS required fewer federal monitoring surveys to be standard surveys and allowed more monitoring surveys to be the narrower scoped and less-resource intensive revisits and complaint investigations.[43]
- Special Focus Facilities: CMS reduced the number of nursing homes participating in the SFF program.[44] In 2013, CMS began to reduce the number of homes in the program by instructing states to terminate homes that had been in the program for 18 months without improvement from participating in Medicare and Medicaid. As we have previously reported, between 2013 and 2014, the number of nursing homes in the SFF program dropped by more than half—from 152 to 62. In 2014, CMS began the process of re-building the number of facilities in the SFF program; however, according to CMS officials, the process would be slow, and as of August 2018 there were 85 SFFs.

In 2015, CMS said some of the reductions to oversight activities were in response to an increase in oversight responsibilities and limited number of staff and financial resources. Specifically, CMS officials said increasing oversight responsibilities and a limited number of staff and financial resources at the central, regional, and state levels required the agency to evaluate its activities and reduce the scope of some activities. In the October 2015 report, we recommended CMS monitor oversight modifications to better assess their effects; HHS agreed with the

---

[43] Before 2013, CMS required 80 percent of these federal monitoring surveys be standard surveys—the most comprehensive type—which cover a broad range of quality issues within a nursing home. The remaining 20 percent of surveys were permitted to be either revisit or complaint surveys, which are more narrow in scope and are also less-resource intensive.

[44] Nursing homes placed in the SFF program receive additional oversight because of the homes' history of poor performance. If homes do not improve the quality of their care, CMS can terminate their participation in Medicare and Medicaid.

recommendation and told us they are beginning to take steps to address this issue. We maintain the importance of monitoring to help CMS better understand how its oversight modifications affect nursing home quality and to improve its oversight given limited resources.[45]

Chairman Harper, Ranking Member DeGette, and Members of the Subcommittee, this concludes my prepared statement. I would be pleased to respond to any questions that you may have at this time.

Mr. Harper. Thank you, Mr. Dicken.

This is now the members' opportunity to ask questions of each of you to learn more about this very important issue, so I will recognize myself for 5 minutes.

Ms. Dorrill, HHS OIG has identified improving care for vulnerable populations including the care provided to individuals in nursing homes as a top management challenge for a decade. Could you expand on this and tell us why ensuring nursing home residents receive the proper standard of care continues to be such a long-standing challenge for HHS and specifically CMS?

Ms. Dorrill. Yes, thank you for the question. It certainly is true that we have considered this a top management challenge for years and we would love to have that removed from the list. But unfortunately the problems remain. And I think it is important to note that although so many of these problems are longstanding that we are in a different place in time so the heavy lift with revising recommendations that has been done, when I said in my statement that we have a framework I think that's correct. And so we are at a different place than we were when we cited those TMCs over the years.

Mr. Harper. Is that a better place?

Ms. Dorrill. Yes. I think it's a first step, absolutely. And that but the proof will be in the execution of that, that sometimes a requirement and the actions of the homes just like emergency planning can be miles apart. And so, but that first step was an enormous one and an important one. And so

---

[45] Under federal internal control standards, ongoing monitoring should occur in the course of normal program operations. See GAO, *Standards for Internal Control in the Federal Government*, GAO/AIMD-00-21.3.1 (Washington, D.C.: Nov. 1999).

we would hope as we see execution over the next couple of years that we might be able to eliminate this concern from our top management challenges.

Mr. Harper. Do you see now that you and CMS are all on the same page?

Ms. Dorrill. It's a great question, yes and no. Yes, on some factors we feel that in respect to our adverse events the harm from medical care that CMS has been proactive in they pulled us into the process of providing that guidance based on our expertise and have laid out very explicit instructions for nursing homes and surveyors. In other areas I wouldn't grade them as highly.

Mr. Harper. Mr. Dicken, I would like to ask you a similar question. Given GAO's substantial body of work examining Federal efforts related to nursing home quality of care, have any issues stood out to you as being long-term challenges for CMS?

Mr. Dicken. Yes, thank you. And I think as you note that we do have a long-term body of work and many of those same types of issues have occurred. We are pleased that over the years CMS has implemented many of the recommendations we've had and made a number of changes. Certainly we've seen improvements in things like training of surveyors, a more standardized methodology for surveyors. We do continue to see that there's important need to make sure that information that CMS is receiving is accurate and that they're using it for assessing States consistently.

And very important that as there are a number of changes occurring over the years that CMS and others continue to monitor to see what the effects of those changes actually are, both in some of the improvements and the enhancements that have been made as well as some of the reductions in oversight that have been made.

Mr. Harper. All right. Let me just follow up on that just a little bit if I can. Are there any aspects of CMS' efforts relating to nursing homes that GAO's work may have touched on would you believe merit additional attention?

Mr. Dicken. Well, we do still have a number of open recommendations that CMS has taken some steps in, one, in trying to make sure the information's more accurate. I think Dr. Goodrich mentioned that they have now much more verifiable information on staffing and are using that to more thoroughly look at and use inspections of staffing.

There are other areas still, however, where they still need to make sure that getting accurate information and of monitoring those effects.

Mr. Harper. And, Dr. Goodrich, if I can ask you a question. Obviously in my opening statement I mentioned the terrible tragedy in Florida at Hollywood Hills at the Rehabilitation Center. And I know CMS terminated the facility from Medicare and Medicaid and has obviously recognized how horrible that is.

The owner of the facility still has an ownership interest in 11 other facilities. Under CMS' current authority, is there anything preventing him from opening a new or additional nursing home facility?

Dr. Goodrich. So thank you for the question. The tragedy at Hollywood Hills was just that, devastating tragedy that should never have happened. As has been said before, it was a complete management failure. As I understand the facts of this case, there's nothing in Medicare that prevents Dr. Michel—if I'm saying his name right——

Mr. Harper. Yes.

Dr. Goodrich [continuing]. From having ownership interest in Medicare facilities. Medicare can only bar an individual who has been convicted of a felony or who is on the OIG exclusion list.

Mr. Harper. In light of Dr. Michel's history, do you believe you need additional tools that can restrict based upon something less than a criminal conviction?

Dr. Goodrich. So this is not my exact area, but I am aware that CMS issued a proposed rule in 2016 to further enhance our program integrity abilities related to this area. We received a number of comments on that rule and we are currently considering them in terms of how to move forward.

Mr. Harper. Thank you, Dr. Goodrich.

The chair will now recognize Ranking Member DeGette for 5 minutes.

Ms. DeGette. Thank you.

Ms. Dorrill mentioned that updating the recommendations is going to be the first step to trying to solve this problem. And as I mentioned in my opening statement, in 2016 CMS issued regulations that updated the Federal health and safety rules for nursing homes.

I know, Dr. Goodrich, that CMS is now in the process of implementing those regulations. I think the one you just referred to is probably one of them. You said that in your testimony these changes are the first comprehensive updates of the nursing home regulations since 1991; is that right? Yes Dr. Goodrich.

Dr. Goodrich. Sorry. That is correct.

Ms. DeGette. And so I am assuming that a lot has changed in the industry that would necessitate an update to those rules and I would assume that the 2016 regulations were designed in part to reflect the advancements and improve how the industry provides quality care to nursing home residents; is that correct?

Dr. Goodrich. Yes, that is correct.

Ms. DeGette. And as I said in my opening statement, since the rules have been finalized CMS has taken several actions that could delay some of them or roll them back altogether. First of all, the rules were designed to be implemented in phases, but not all the phases have been implemented yet.

Second, CMS now has issued a moratorium on enforcing some of those rules, and, finally, last year CMS launched a review of nursing home regulations to or requirements to determine whether any of them placed procedural burdens on facilities. So it sounds like maybe some of these proposed rules will never be implemented; is that correct?

Dr. Goodrich. We are currently in the process as you mentioned of implementing the rule that we finalized in 2016. We are on target for implementing all three of the phases and that is underway now.

Ms. DeGette. OK. And what is your timeframe for implementing all of the phases?

Dr. Goodrich. So phase 1 was implemented shortly after the publication of the final rule in 2016. This was really the things that nursing homes were already doing or were very simple to achieve.

Ms. DeGette. OK.

Dr. Goodrich. Phase 2, we began implementation and surveying and enforcing on November 28th of 2017, so that is underway now. We've surveyed about——

Ms. DeGette. It has been about a year.

Dr. Goodrich. It's been about a year and phase 3 begins in November of 2019.

Ms. DeGette. And how long will that take?

Dr. Goodrich. So nursing homes are expected to be compliant with the phase 3 requirements by November of 2019. So at that time that will be the expectation.

Ms. DeGette. OK. And so let me just ask the question again. Do you anticipate that all of the 2016 rules will be implemented?

Dr. Goodrich. Yes, we are on track to implement the 2016 final rule.

Ms. DeGette. OK. Now I want to ask you a question about a CMS proposal that might prohibit nursing home residents from being able to bring a lawsuit. There is a rule that bans pre-dispute arbitration agreements and CMS has signaled it may remove it. In other words CMS is proposing to remove what I consider to be a consumer protection rule that was designed to make sure that nursing home residents could go to court or could join other people in lawsuits to settle grievances and that they wouldn't be forced into arbitration.

I know a lot of groups like the AARP have expressed concerns about this proposed change. What is the status of that? Does CMS intend to do that and why?

Dr. Goodrich. So as you mentioned as part of the 2016 final rule we did impose a ban on pre-dispute arbitration.

Ms. DeGette. Yes.

Dr. Goodrich. Shortly thereafter, Department of Health and Human Services was sued for an injunction, a preliminary and permanent injunction to stop CMS from enforcing that ban on pre-dispute arbitration. The court granted a preliminary injunction in November of 2016, so we currently cannot enforce what we finalized——

Ms. DeGette. Did by court order?

Dr. Goodrich. Yes.

Ms. DeGette. And what is the status of that lawsuit, do you know?

Dr. Goodrich. I'm not certain of the status but the injunction is still in place so we are not able to enforce.

Ms. DeGette. If you could get us the status of that lawsuit that would be——

Dr. Goodrich. Certainly.

Ms. DeGette [continuing]. Very helpful to us because my view and I think Congresswoman Schakowsky would really agree with me about this as one of the most effective ways to address if we see rampant nursing home abuses is when patients can bring class actions against some of these bad actors. And, you know, these families they are going into nursing homes, they are being asked to sign these arbitration agreements. They are so desperate to get the health—as I think all of you have said, these are families in crisis many times and so they just sign it and then they have signed away their legal rights.

So we will do everything we can, I think, to make sure that we can enforce that 2016 rule that people don't have to be forced to sign arbitration agreements. With that I yield back.

Mr. Harper. The gentlewoman yields back.

The chair will now recognize the gentleman from Oregon, the chair of the full committee, Mr. Walden, for 5 minutes.

Mr. Walden. Thank you, Mr. Chairman. And I want to thank our witnesses. We have another hearing going on downstairs and so some of us have to bounce back and forth.

Dr. Goodrich, a September 2017 data brief issued by the OIG indicated that there was a significant amount of variation with respect to how state survey agencies classified the complaints they received. For example, data compiled by the OIG showed that in 2015 there were three States that prioritized complaints as being immediate jeopardy at least 40 percent of the time, while eight States did not designate any of their complaints as immediate jeopardy.

Can you explain why there seems to be such a variation in how States prioritize complaints and what is CMS doing to ensure that complaints and deficiencies are addressed in a more consistent manner?

Dr. Goodrich. Yes, thank you for the question. So, first, I want to say we very much appreciate the work of the OIG and the GAO in the oversight of our programs. They really help to make our programs better and we have concurred with the vast majority of their recommendations particularly on this issue around state service oversight, state agency oversight.

So we are undertaking actively a number of actions to address exactly these recommendations. So number one, CMS regional offices do meet quarterly with the state survey agencies to discuss issues, look at trends and how they're performing, any concerns that they may have. We also recently undertook an effort to really overhaul our Federal oversight surveys.

We are required to conduct Federal oversight surveys of about five percent of state surveys or at least five state surveys and we've been doing this for awhile, but we've undertaken an effort beginning in April of this year to revise that process in response to what we learned from the OIG as well as the GAO. So that's underway now as well.

We also give monthly feedback reports to the state survey agencies that we began in April of this year which allow them to understand where their own deficiencies are, where there may be patterns of inconsistencies or where they're not appropriately citing deficiencies as they should. And this has really been made possible by the new standardized software-based survey process that we implemented last fall across the country.

Mr. Walden. Ah, OK.

Dr. Goodrich. And then finally we are in the process right now of really overhauling the State Performance Standards System. This is a system that we've had underway for awhile, but again in response to the recommendations from the OIG and the GAO we began an effort again in April of this year to evaluate this entire program to identify ways to improve it. It's a very large-scale effort, will take at least a year to do but is well underway. And it's really focused on improving the efficiency and the effectiveness of measuring and improving state performance.

Mr. Walden. Right.

Dr. Goodrich. So we're very happy that we have these recommendations and that we're moving forward on them.

Mr. Walden. Good, thank you. Admittedly, this is old, but my mother spent her last few months in a nursing home in our hometown 28 years ago. And I spent a lot of time in and out as you do with a parent and I was always struck by how much time the people that were giving health care had to spend on paperwork. And they would be off in the cafeteria and I went over, and I was in state legislature at the time, and I said what is all this, and just reams of paper, paper, paper.

And I thought at some point, here, as public policy people we want what everybody wants is quality safe care especially for this vulnerable and difficult fragile population and sometimes government just overreacts and says we need a new rule, we need a new regulation, we need another something which in the end eats up the resource that is hard to get.

It is hard to, as we all know there are medical shortages in terms of nurses and aides and everybody else and it just struck me that would my mother have been better off with less reporting and paperwork and somebody that actually was checking on her more often. Do you know what I mean? And we have got to have both, it is finding this right balance. But boy, I hope somebody is looking at just the layer, a layer, a layer we tend to add on to address a single problem that may occur in Florida and so we think we have to do this everywhere.

And looks at are there some things that we could peel back that would actually allow improved quality of care and then what are the real management tools we need and make sure they are being enforced effectively in this process. It is hard, I know, but I have seen it firsthand. My parents, both my parents and my mother-in- law and over the years and, you know, you realize it is a difficult population and very fragile medically. Things happen and mistakes are made and there are some bad actors.

And so I just hope as you all are doing your work somebody is looking at that angle as well so the measrements and the tools for enforcement are effective but make sense too. So, Mr. Chairman, I yield back.

Mr. Harper. The gentleman yields back. The chair will now recognize the gentlewoman from Florida, Ms. Castor, for 5 minutes.

Ms. Castor. Thank you, Mr. Chairman. I think this investigation by the committee is very important on nursing home resident care and the quality of our skilled nursing centers across the country and I appreciate the focus on emergency preparedness. It has not been a year since Hurricane Irma swept through and I think it is important for us to go through what CMS is doing, what States are doing.

One thing that should not be done has become clear here as was reported by the AP earlier this year. As Hurricane Irma bore down on Florida, Governor Rick Scott gave out his cell phone number during a conference call with administrators of the State's nursing homes and assisted living facilities. He told them to contact him if they ran into problems and he would try to get help.

So they did 120 times according to phone records released earlier this year, not last year. Nearly all the calls went directly to voice mail before being returned. The Associated Press reached 29 of the callers and found that in numerous cases the Governor's offer to personally intervene may have slowed efforts to get help and fostered unrealistic and potentially dangerous expectations that Scott could resolve problems.

Irma knocked out power across much of Florida as its strongest winds swept from Key West to Jacksonville, so most of the skilled nursing centers asked for restoration of electricity. But Florida is served by private electric companies and municipal utilities and none are directed by the state, so the Governor's office could only request that particular nursing homes be given priority.

Twelve patients later died of overheating at a nursing home that called Scott's cell phone three times. Its administrators say Scott's staff didn't get them help restoring the air conditioning but we know it was a significant management failure as well by the owners of Hollywood Hills. This cannot be the answer for emergency preparedness.

So I understand now there are new requirements that went into effect in November of 2016. CMS is now surveying states. That began last year. What have we found? Are the states following through? I will let you begin, Doctor.

Dr. Goodrich. Absolutely. Thank you for the question. As you mentioned, we did finalize the emergency preparedness rule in November of 2016. This applied to all Medicare-certified facilities certainly including long-term care facilities or nursing homes. We began verifying that compliance in November of 2017.

So far we have surveyed about 75 percent of facilities. We anticipate we will have surveyed across the country a hundred percent of facilities by February of 2019. As you noted, there is a need for proper communications systems when there is a disaster and one of the components of the emergency preparedness rule that facilities are now required to adhere to is to develop and maintain communications systems to contact appropriate staff and authorities.

Ms. Castor. So are you finding now in the surveys that they are adhering to the new requirements?

Dr. Goodrich. So we are finding currently that there have been some providers that have been cited for noncompliance so we are working with them to bring them into compliance rapidly. That is an area that they are required to adhere to. Currently, we are not finding that that is one of the most commonly cited deficiencies, but it is something that we are surveying for actively.

Ms. Castor. Thank you. States have a critical role here and I am concerned with certain States not following through with requirements. For instance, OIG's audits have found that some States fell short in investigating the most serious complaints in nursing homes.

Ms. Dorrill, what are the nature of these complaints and what should we expect the States to do in response?

Ms. Dorrill. The complaints ran across the board and then half of them were associated with high priority or immediate jeopardy, so serious complaints. And so I think the issue at hand is that states have to be held accountable. Dr. Goodrich talked a bit about that system and I think it's critical to all these pieces coming together that the states are understanding the new requirements and effectively enforcing those in the homes.

Ms. Castor. Do you believe CMS is holding states accountable when they do not follow through with their responsibilities?

Ms. Dorrill. So much of this is new, we'll certainly be looking at it. But so much of the new requirement in the guidance is just new within the last 9 months and so we don't know but we certainly have pointed out weaknesses. And we think that it's a two-pronged approach. It's education and it's also ensuring that there's some kind of accountability on the part of the States to ensure that they follow through.

Ms. Castor. Thank you. I yield back.

Mr. Harper. The gentlewoman yields back. The chair will now recognize the gentleman from Virginia, the vice chairman of the subcommittee, for 5 minutes.

Mr. Griffith. Thank you very much, Mr. Chairman. I greatly appreciate it.

Dr. Goodrich, my colleagues, Congresswoman Black, Congressman Adrian Smith, Luja´ n, and Crowley and I recently introduced the Reducing Unnecessary Senior Hospitalization Act of 2018 which seeks to improve quality in nursing homes by providing quality acute care at patients' bedsides via telehealth instead of transferring them to the hospital. By CMS' own calculations, two- thirds of hospital transfers are avoidable leading to increased costs to Medicare and negatively impacting health outcomes and quality of care.

What are your thoughts on the potential for complementing current nursing home staff with emergency trained first responders utilizing telehealth to connect physician specialists, i.e., emergency physicians that might not otherwise be available to this patient population?

Dr. Goodrich. So thank you for that question and letting me know about this pending legislation. So we do understand that as you mentioned transfers to the hospital, that's a very disrupting event for a nursing home patient and many of them are avoidable. This is something we actually measure as part of our quality reporting programs so we're certainly aware that there's a significant level of admissions to a hospital.

So we would be very interested and willing to provide technical assistance to you and your staff on this legislation at your convenience.

Mr. Griffith. Well, I appreciate that very much and thank you. I am really excited by telemedicine. Representing a fairly rural district, I can tell you that one of my small nursing home chains has implemented wound care by using telemedicine, so they have a wound care specialist who is available.

And one of their nurses will go in and see the patient who may have a bedsore or some other kind of injury and they are looking at through a pair of glasses that has a camera on it and the wound specialist wherever they are in the United States can see that wound, get a color picture, be able then to tell the nursing home staff what needs to be done to make sure that that wound is being treated properly and taken care of. So I am really excited about telemedicine as a whole.

Let me go to your payroll-based journal for staffing, because I do think that sometimes there may be some confusion. And while we recognize that we want the staffing to be there so you all can use it as a tool, you mentioned it in your statement, Mr. Dicken mentioned in his that the self-reporting hadn't worked because there was a difference.

But I think that may be a little unfair to CMS and to the nursing homes affected, to some of them. Not the bad actors but people that are really trying, because am I not correct that it is a slightly different standard? In self-reporting if you had a salaried employee who worked 50–55 hours a week they got to count that extra time, but under your report which I have no quarrel with, I am just saying they are different, you only count those folks at a maximum of 40 hours of being on the floor.

Likewise, if you have an LPN who is doing supervisory work, they don't get credit for their supervisory time where an RN would. Again no quarrel with the change, but just saying that to say that the old reporting system was intentionally underreporting might not be fair since it is really apples to oranges. Wouldn't you agree with that?

Dr. Goodrich. The previous reporting system was essentially a 2-week snapshot that the nursing homes completed on a form during their recertification survey. The current system as you mentioned is based upon daily staffing levels of numerous different types of staff that the nursing homes have to report quarterly to CMS. And certainly as we were standing that up we had to make certain decisions around ensuring that what is reported is auditable back to the payroll so that it could be as it is required by law so that it could be as accurate as possible.

So the situations you mentioned around a salaried employee, yes, we only count the 40 hours a week that they would be working.

Mr. Griffith. And I don't have any quarrel with that but to say that there was understaffing previously when you are using different metrics wouldn't really be fair to CMS or to some of the nursing homes. Wouldn't that be fair to say?

Dr. Goodrich. I would say it's very difficult to compare the two.

Mr. Griffith. Difficult to compare, OK.

The Commonwealth of Virginia partnering with healthcare providers developed a long-term care mutual aid plan which is a voluntary agreement among participating nursing homes that they will share supplies, resources, and house residents from other facilities if a serious need arises. We heard Chairman Walden say earlier that one of his nursing homes or a small chain had a facility in California and was looking to move patients to Oregon. This is actually a statewide system.

Are you familiar with this type of plan and do you think it will work and do you think other sStates will adopt it?

Dr. Goodrich. I am not familiar with this kind of plan but we certainly would be interested to learn more and again our staff would be glad to follow up with you on this.

Mr. Griffith. Very good. Thank you so much.

I yield back, Mr. Chairman.

Mr. Harper. The gentleman yields back. The chair will now recognize the gentleman from California, Mr. Ruiz, for 5 minutes.

Mr. Ruiz. Thank you, Mr. Chairman. Taking care of seniors has been a big priority for me as a physician. I am an emergency medicine doctor, Dr. Goodrich, and now as a Member of Congress advocating for them here. And when a loved one is placed in the care of a nursing home, we trust and expect that they will receive high quality care and as we know many nursing homes do exactly that. But it is also clear from years of reports from OIG and GAO that there are problematic providers out there.

Ms. Dorrill, your office did groundbreaking work that identified instances of adverse events in nursing homes and you found that one in three Medicare beneficiaries experienced harm during their stay. So what kind of adverse events did these residents experience, can you elaborate on those?

Ms. Dorrill. Yes, thank you for the question. It really ranged the gamut. And that's actually a part of our message is that we found that nursing homes were focusing on just a small number of events, falls with injury, for example, and pressure ulcers, and they were excluding a broad range of events that were already happening that went unnoticed as harm. Things like blood clots and dehydration that can seem like subtle——

Mr. Ruiz. That they didn't identify and allowed it to persist for a time. How about medical errors, giving the wrong medication, et cetera?

Ms. Dorrill. Fourteen percent of our events involve medical error. When a lot of people think about adverse events they think it's all medical error. But one of the things that we've tried to promulgate is this notion that adverse events can occur from general substandard care. It's not really a mistake, it's just not doing the right thing.

Mr. Ruiz. So you say that half of these were preventable. Can you give me some examples of those that were not preventable that——

Ms. Dorrill. Yes. So, for example, if someone was given a medication and they were allergic to that and had a reaction but no one knew that they were allergic, that was not information that the physician could have acted upon.

Mr. Ruiz. And so are these different adverse events not on the state agencies' survey lists? Why are they not looking for these?

Ms. Dorrill. I think that there's been a revolution and this is true for hospitals too in the whole notion of adverse events. And CMS has changed its hospitals provisions as well that I think there was just a narrow focus on a small number of events and people weren't thinking about harm more broadly.

Mr. Ruiz. So they weren't.

Ms. Dorrill. No.

Mr. Ruiz. They weren't looking for these different types of adverse events.

Ms. Dorrill. That's correct.

Mr. Ruiz. So I would like to turn to another quality of care concern. In your recent reporting, OIG again identified Medicare beneficiaries in nursing homes who suffered harm, this time from abuse and neglect, where still OIG found that, quote, a significant percentage of these incidents may not have been reported to law enforcement.

So I find this very troubling and so did you, or OIG, enough to issue an early alert to CMS about the findings. What are some of the immediate actions CMS can take to address these vulnerabilities?

Ms. Dorrill. Thank you. We first requested that they do what we did which is it's possible to look in the claims and find out a lot of these things are claims associated with abuse and neglect and that we suggested that CMS do that to monitor the situation. And then, secondly, we also suggested that they enhance their pursuit of the authority to be able to give remedies when these events were not reported.

Mr. Ruiz. Dr. Goodrich, what has the agency taken, what actions has the agency taken to address this finding?

Dr. Goodrich. So regarding the recommendation to look in the claims for emergency room services and matching those claims to skilled nursing facilities, that is something that we are currently exploring the feasibility of doing.

Mr. Ruiz. You haven't started it but you are just looking into it.

Dr. Goodrich. We're exploring whether or not that's feasible to do to be able to have that information to the surveyors.

Mr. Ruiz. Well, by law, as an emergency physician if somebody reports any suspicion of abuse or neglect that has to go into the medical record and that has to be reported to the county officials and APS and all that so that would be a good place to start.

I have another question in terms of empowering the clients and consumers and also their families. Is there any requirement that when a patient gets or a person gets admitted to a nursing home during the orientation that they are given an understanding of their rights, of quality measures, resources, to understand more about what those quality measures are and also a way to report any concerns to a third party like an agency or CMS, is that a requirement, part of your requirements for CMS so that they know that and is that being implemented properly?

Dr. Goodrich. Yes. So yes, that is a requirement as part of our requirements for participation that residents or their, and their families or their surrogates be informed of their rights as soon as they are admitted into a nursing facility and that they are informed of their rights to file complaints with the state survey agency or with law enforcement.

Mr. Ruiz. Are they given the information on how to do that?

Dr. Goodrich. Yes, it's supposed to be posted in the nursing home. Sorry, I'm not familiar with the details.

Mr. Ruiz. Yes, see, that is the difference that Ms. Dorrill was saying. It is either posted or you have something in writing, but the true understanding and the implementation of that information is a different story.

So do we know if it is being conducted in a way where during the orientation they are being explained on how to file a complaint?

Dr. Goodrich. Yes. As part of the admission process in addition to everything about the plan of care in clinical care, one of our conditions or requirements for participation is around patient rights and being informed of those rights.

Mr. Ruiz. Thank you.

Mr. Harper. The gentleman yields back. The chair will now recognize the gentlewoman from Indiana, Mrs. Brooks, for 5 minutes.

Mrs. Brooks. Thank you, Mr. Chairman, and thank you for holding this very important hearing.

Ms. Dorrill, I would like, as Chairman Harper talked about in his opening statement, I want to focus a little bit on my line of questioning regarding the owner of the facility where the 12 residents died in the aftermath of Hurricane Irma, the Hollywood Hills. Because it is my understanding that Dr. Michel had been the subject of wrongdoing in the past, including settling with the Department of Justice long ago, corporate integrity agreement, after being implicated in a scheme to receive kickbacks for providing unnecessary medical treatment to elderly residents, and that was the '06 timeframe.

Can you please explain—and I am a former U.S. Attorney so I have worked with HHS OIG. Can you explain what tools are available to you to exclude facility owners from owning nursing homes if obviously OIG had determined and there was a settlement and so forth, but they were involved in participating in this unlawful conduct or fraud, can you go into deeper detail about exclusion process?

Ms. Dorrill. Yes, just to say though, I'm not in the Counsel's Office. I'm not an investigator but I'll do my best, that OIG has a number of tools at our disposal and this it's critical to us. It's the main part of our work that we hold wrongdoers accountable. And so I think the important thing to remember is that those tools are at our disposal and that it depends on the specific facts and circumstances of the case what direction we go.

But we certainly have the exclusion authority. We also have tools such as under the False Claims Act we have the ability to impose civil monetary penalties. We also have hundreds of criminal investigators who help their law enforcement partners to investigate criminal cases. So it's a broad range of activity and core to our mission.

Mrs. Brooks. Can you talk a little bit though about the exclusion authority tool and how long the process takes, who ultimately makes the decision as to when a provider is on the exclusion list?

Ms. Dorrill. So for those who may not be familiar, and again I'm not in the Counsel's Office, but the OIG can exclude individuals and entities from Federal programs such as Medicare and Medicaid for various types of conduct set forth in statute, including false claims. The primary effect of that exclusion is it will no longer pay for services and we maintain a database with all that information publicly.

OIG has certainly excluded nursing home providers. We recently excluded a 13-facility nursing home chain. We have something like 70,000 excluded providers now, something like 1,600 just this fiscal year alone. So I don't know if that fully answers your question.

Mrs. Brooks. It doesn't require though a criminal conviction then for a person to be excluded or an entity to be excluded?

Ms. Dorrill. I'll need to take that question, I'd be so happy to, back to my Counsel's Office to make sure that I can give you accurate information there.

Mrs. Brooks. I think we would like to know more information about the exclusion process from Counsel's Office and from your office particularly relative to, not only we had that incident, but as I understand there are other incidents involving this particular provider let alone the Hollywood Hills incident. So I am interested in knowing how long the process takes, who makes the final decisions, what are the categories that a person can be excluded.

Then I would like to ask both you and Dr. Goodrich a little bit more about the emergency preparedness issues. We are reauthorizing what is called PAHPA, Pandemic All-Hazards Preparedness Act, and we are including in that a provision to have the National Academy of Medicine do an overview of emergency preparedness by hospitals but also long-term care facilities. And because as I am hearing you both say that while there might be plans in place that doesn't necessarily mean the execution of those plans happen.

And do you believe there needs to be more attention to this emergency preparedness that we are not doing enough? Dr. Goodrich?

Dr. Goodrich. Thank you. Obviously this is a huge priority for us especially given the events of last year. So as we've mentioned we are in the process, in the early process of implementing that regulation and surveying facilities for that. So as you're working, doing your work on this area we'd be more than happy to give you technical assistance and talk through these issues with you. But we are early in the process and I think learning how it is going.

Mrs. Brooks. OK, thank you.

Ms. Dorrill, anything further before my time is expired?

Ms. Dorrill. No, just asserting that we found significant problems with the emergency planning and appreciate your focus on that area.

Mrs. Brooks. Thank you. I yield back.

Mr. Harper. The gentlewoman yields back. The chair will now recognize the gentlewoman from Illinois, Ms. Schakowsky, for 5 minutes.

Ms. Schakowsky. Thank you, Mr. Chairman.

If I sound a little impatient about this focus on nursing home and safety it is because I have been working on this issue since the mid-80s, including when I was in the state legislature in Illinois and ever since I have been here in Congress. There are some provisions in the Affordable Care Act that deal with nursing homes that I was successful in getting into the legislation. But I don't know how many GAO reports there have been. I don't know how many reports from oversight committees there have been about these persistent problems.

And as we enter into this age where more, the aging of America, the graying of America, more and more people needing long-term care including nursing homes, it is hard for me to hear words like, this is an important first step. I mean we need to be making last steps now. We need to be getting at the heart of the problem.

Let me ask you, Dr. Goodrich, who has the primary responsibility to make sure that nursing home quality standards are met, States or CMS? And is it the policy of the Trump administration to shift more of the responsibility to the States?

Dr. Goodrich. So it is a shared responsibility between the States and CMS. We promulgate the regulations and then we oversee the state survey agencies in their implementation of the surveys of the nursing homes and the implementation of those regulations. And as I——

Ms. Schakowsky. Are we seeing more of a shift toward States or is this always standard?

Dr. Goodrich. Our process for overseeing health and safety for nursing homes remains the same. It hasn't changed. It remains a partnership in the way that I just described.

Ms. Schakowsky. What was the rationale behind no longer imposing financial penalties for each day of a violation? Couldn't that be seen as a weakening of a commitment to enforcement?

Dr. Goodrich. Specifically related to the civil monetary penalties what we were seeing over the last few years and what had been, I think, also recognized by others was that there was quite a bit of variation in how civil monetary penalties were being applied across the country. In some areas not being applied enough when they should have been and in other areas being applied in situations when actually should have had different enforcement remedies applied.

So we sought to make that process more standardized and more uniform so that there was consistency across the country in the correct application of civil monetary penalties. And so last year what we did was we worked with the regional offices and we developed a civil monetary penalty tool so that survey agencies and our regional offices could go and use that tool which has essentially an algorithm in it to ensure that regions are consistently and accurately applying civil monetary penalties.

Ms. Schakowsky. Except that I am asking about the penalties then, not the monitoring, the penalties, no longer imposing financial penalties for each day.

Dr. Goodrich. So we do still impose financial penalties for each day, so per day penalties depending upon the circumstance. And the number of those penalties has actually risen over the last 4 years. In 2014 we had just over 1,100 per day civil monetary penalties and in 2017 we had almost 2,000 per day.

Ms. Schakowsky. So let me ask you this. Do the nursing home advocates support these changes?

Dr. Goodrich. We have certainly worked with and been transparent about our intents here related to——

Ms. Schakowsky. That is kind of a yes or no.

Dr. Goodrich. I would have to ask the nursing home advocates. We certainly have had discussions with them about this. We have seen——

Ms. Schakowsky. My understanding is no. Let me also, I want to get to a Human Rights Watch report[46] found that in an average week nursing facilities in the United States administer powerful anti-psychotropic drugs

---

[46] The information has been retained in committee files and can be found at: https://docs.house.gov/meetings/IF/IF02/20180906/108648/HHRG-115-IF02-20180906-SD003.pdf.

in over 179,000 people who don't need them. I ask unanimous consent to enter that report into the record.

Mr. Harper. Without objection.

[The information appears at the conclusion of the hearing.]

Ms. Schakowsky. These drugs are often given without informed consent. This is after a 2011 OIG report that found rampant over-use of these anti-psychotic drugs.

So, Dr. Goodrich, what actions are CMS taking to address the high rate of these drugs and used 7 years after that OIG report?

Dr. Goodrich. So we would completely agree that this has been a very significant quality and safety issue within nursing homes. That is why in 2011 in partnership with a number of stakeholders we launched the National Partnership to Improve Dementia Care in Nursing Homes, which was a holistic effort around dementia care, but definitely had a very serious focus around reducing inappropriate use of anti-psychotics in nursing homes.

We have seen over that time period from 2011 to early 2017 a 34 percent reduction in the inappropriate use of anti-psychotics and we are now focusing——

Ms. Schakowsky. So two-thirds still remains.

Dr. Goodrich. So there is still overuse. That is true. And there are particular nursing homes in the country who have not made the kinds of improvements that we would hope. And so we have set a new goal to focus on those facilities that are still overusing to unacceptable extent.

Ms. Schakowsky. Thank you.

Mr. Harper. The gentlewoman yields back. The chair will now recognize the gentlewoman from California, Mrs. Walters, for 5 minutes.

Mrs. Walters. Thank you, Mr. Chairman. Federal regulations enumerate a limited number of circumstances under which a nursing facility or skilled nursing facility may transfer or discharge a resident against their will. Under Federal law, a nursing facility or skilled nursing facility must also readmit residents who may temporarily leave for a hospitalization. However, claims that nursing home residents are being dumped or denied readmission appears to be a growing concern.

For example, according to press reports, the California State Long-term Care Ombudsman received more than 1,500 complaints in 2016 alleging that residents have been improperly discharged or evicted from nursing homes in California. This is a 73 percent increase from the number of complaints received since 2011. The Illinois State Ombudsman has stated that such complaints have more than doubled since 2011.

Dr. Goodrich, does CMS view involuntary discharges of nursing home residents or denials of readmission as a significant problem?

Dr. Goodrich. Yes. This is something that we have also heard reports about happening and it is something that we're concerned about absolutely.

Mrs. Walters. When nursing home residents are involuntarily discharged from or denied readmission to a nursing home after a hospital stay, where do they typically end up and how are they cared for?

Dr. Goodrich. So I think that's variable and that is something that we are trying to explore a little further to understand what's happening on the ground with these residents. So certainly where they end up if that's your question can be quite variable. It can be, with a family member and another facility is often where they will end up going as well.

Mrs. Walters. Are you guys trying to do any sort of analysis on this to find out exactly where they are ending up?

Dr. Goodrich. I'd be happy to get back to you with the answer to the question to how we're taking a look at that. I'm not sure of the specifics.

Mrs. Walters. Did you want to add something?

Ms. Dorrill. We have, we're currently underway on this exact issue. I share your concern and we have a study that will be coming out shortly that will be of interest to you.

Mrs. Walters. OK, thank you.

Federal law also requires States provide nursing home residents, who allege they were improperly discharged or transferred, with a hearing and, if appropriate, provide for residents a readmission to the nursing home if they prevail. However, it has been alleged that California is failing to enforce its own hearing decisions in instances where decisions have been rendered in favor of residents.

In a 2012 letter to the California Department of Public Health, Center for Healthcare Quality, CMS stated that while it could not advise California what particular state agency should enforce the hearing decisions, as that is for the States to decide, CMS regulations are clear that the state agency must promptly make corrective actions. CMS reiterated California's obligation to enforce its hearing decisions in a letter sent on August 31st, 2017.

Dr. Goodrich, how does CMS verify that States are fulfilling their legal obligations to adjudicate and enforce hearing decisions related to improper nurse home discharges or transfers?

Dr. Goodrich. So this is a topic with which I'm not terribly familiar of the specifics of the California case, but we'd be very happy to take a look at it and get back to you with responses to that.

Mrs. Walters. OK, so then I don't know if you can answer these two questions but I will ask you. Does CMS know whether California is meeting its legal obligations to enforce these decisions?

Dr. Goodrich. I'm not personally aware but we will get back to you with that.

Mrs. Walters. OK, then I have one more. Does CMS know of or have reason to believe other States may be failing to enforce their hearing decisions?

Dr. Goodrich. I think that's something we certainly would be concerned about and would be happy to get back to you with responses.

Mrs. Walters. OK, if you guys could follow up——

Dr. Goodrich. We will.

Mrs. Walters [continuing]. And get back to the committee on that we would really appreciate it.

Dr. Goodrich. Of course.

Mrs. Walters. Thank you and I yield back the balance of my time.

Mr. Harper. The gentlewoman yields back. I will now recognize the vice chairman of the subcommittee, Mr. Griffith, for the purposes of a follow-up question.

Mr. Griffith. Yes, and I think that Ms. Schakowsky and I might be on the same side, we might not be, but it deals with the daily fines and so forth. Because I am aware of a situation, so I am glad you are looking at it so we can get these algorithms where they make sense because you want to punish people for bad acts.

But I am aware of a situation where coffee was spilled. There was an incident. Something should have been said but somehow the fine ended up being between $1 million and $2 million dollars. The patient never went to the hospital. No serious injuries. Clearly something needed to be done, but it seemed that maybe the old algorithm was a little out of whack if you end up with a $1 million to $2 million dollar penalty for spilled coffee and no hospitalization.

Dr. Goodrich. So I'm not familiar with that particular incident, but I think that is potentially an example where there was again as I mentioned before we weren't always seeing consistent application of the civil monetary penalties in both directions. And so that's why we really have been trying to standardize that.

Mr. Griffith. And I appreciate that and hope that you all get that all worked out, but agree that there ought to be penalties and there ought to be something that the nursing homes can know that this is what we are supposed to do, and if there is a problem the penalty will be something that is equal to or in the vein of what ought to be happening.

Thank you, yield back.

Mr. Harper. The chair will now recognize Ms. Schakowsky for the purposes of a follow-up question.

Ms. Schakowsky. So in terms of CMS enforcement I wondered how you are using these new—we have been talking somewhat about the payroll staffing data reported by nursing homes to enforce the requirements that each facility have a registered nurse on duty at least 8 hours every day. Let me just state my preference. I think most people who put a person in a nursing home would be shocked that there is not a nurse, a registered nurse 24/7, when they get the bill for the month that there is not a nurse there.

I have a piece of legislation I have introduced, Put a Nurse in a Nursing Home. But I am just wondering how you are following up on that.

Dr. Goodrich. Absolutely. Thank you for bringing that up. We would agree that the new payroll-based journal system gives us really unprecedented insight into staffing within nursing homes. And as you mentioned, some of the things that we have discovered since we started requiring the reporting of those data is exactly what you mentioned, is that there are some nursing homes that do not have a registered nurse as required by our regulations for 8 hours a day, 7 days a week.

And I think even more concerning is that we see fluctuations in some nursing homes, again a minority but it's there, where that those deficiencies in nurse staffing are more common on the weekends than they are on the weekdays. And I can't think of any clinical reason why that should be different on a Saturday than on a Tuesday.

So that is something that we are concerned about and right now we're taking two actions related to that. I will caveat that by saying this is early, we're exploring the data and we're thinking ahead about other ways in which we can use these data better. So number one, one thing we have already done is in the five-star rating system nursing homes that do not have nurse staffing as appropriate for at least 7 days out of a quarter, their star rating goes down to one star and that affects the staffing star rating and that affects that overall star rating as well.

We are also looking at ways in which we could incorporate the findings that I just mentioned about the fluctuations and the lack of nursing as required by regulation further into the star rating system. The second thing that we're doing is we are embedding the data, the staffing data into our survey software which will then allow the state surveyors when they go onsite to do their investigations to have that information around staffing for that nursing home that they are in so that they can look for quality issues that may be related to staffing based upon the data they have right there in their hand.

So those are two ways in which we're, for now, initially using these data, but we'll continue to explore other ways.

Ms. Schakowsky. OK, and any of the other two witnesses want to say anything on this topic? I don't know.

Ms. Dorrill. I just wanted to say that we have work underway now on the payroll-based journal and we plan to look at the accuracy of the data and CMS' use of it at this early implementation.

Ms. Schakowsky. OK. I would really like to see that after you complete your investigation of that issue. So good, thank you very much. I yield back.

Mr. Harper. The chair will now recognize the gentleman, in celebration of his birthday, the gentleman from Georgia, Mr. Carter.

Mr. Carter. Thank you, Mr. Chairman. I appreciate you sharing that with everyone. And I do appreciate it very much.

Mr. Harper. We didn't ask what year.

Mr. Carter. You can't thank me for that as well, yes.

Well, thank all of you for being here. Full disclosure, I am currently the only pharmacist serving in Congress. Not only am I a pharmacist, but I was also a consultant pharmacist and my expertise and my career was spent in institutional pharmacy in nursing homes. I have gone through Federal inspections, state inspections, so this is something that I am very familiar with.

And I have to tell you I was blessed to be in a number of good nursing homes that provided quality care that really cared about the patients and sometimes I could be frustrated by some of the regulations. And I just want to encourage you, a couple of things. First of all, you know, it is important and it is important to have a registered nurse 8 hours a day. It is important to make sure that rules and regulations are followed, but sometimes we get caught up in the cookie cutter approach that one size fits all.

And I just want to encourage you and I say that because I have seen it firsthand. I have seen how nursing homes struggle and they struggle to find good quality help. They don't pay very high, they can't afford to. It is difficult at times. That is no excuse, you still have to have quality care and as I say I was very blessed to be in facilities that provided quality care.

I think that you have—I am sorry I had another hearing, but we have already talked about the payroll-based journal and about the fact that salaried employees, and trust me, I have seen a salaried, a DNS who has is registered as 40 hours seeing a more 60 or 80 hours a week. So that is kind of a misnomer and I hope you take that into consideration.

And then whenever you are talking about a 30-minute lunch break, I have seen them take 5 minutes to cram something in their mouth and go on and continue on. I have also seen it as you well know, and I know I am the preacher preaching to the choir here, but nursing homes can fall apart quickly. I have been in a nursing home in the morning and it was in top shape and then by the afternoon and just because of the patient population it can really fall apart very quickly.

But anyway, having said that I will tell you that I am concerned particularly the Federal inspectors as it relates to the state inspectors. I have seen the state inspectors sometimes try to do too much because the Federal inspectors are following them. Generally what happens is that you would always know if the fire inspector came and then probably the surveyors, the state surveyors were coming next because the fire inspector would always come first and then the state surveyors would come.

And the Federal surveyors would come after the state surveyors in order to see how well the state surveyors had done and sometimes I felt like they were putting undue pressure on some of the state inspectors. Not that they didn't need it at times, they did, and it is important. It is important to have the checks and balances in that and I understand that.

I wanted to ask you and I will ask Dr. Goodrich, you, this question about some of the potential complexity for providers that have that the regulations. As I understand it, there has been a temporary moratorium placed on some of the 194 regulations as a result of the stakeholder feedback. Just to clarify, how many of the 194 regulations had this moratorium placed on them?

Dr. Goodrich. Eight.

Mr. Carter. Eight of them. And out of those eight did any of those have to do with neglect or with abuse?

Dr. Goodrich. They did not.

Mr. Carter. They did not, OK. Good, they should not and I appreciate that. And, finally, do facilities still have to enforce these eight regulations and have a plan in place to fix them if they are noncompliant?

Dr. Goodrich. Absolutely. That's our expectation, yes.

Mr. Carter. That is your expectation, good. Again you know, I have seen the burden that can be placed on these facilities and again no one is accepting and I am certainly not advocating that they shouldn't have quality care. This is a very feeble, if you will, population that needs this help. But I just want to make sure we have balance here. I want you to understand that I have worked side by side with these people in the nursing homes and they are good people for the most part.

Now, like every profession you have bad actors and you have to get rid of those bad actors and to a certain extent, to a large extent that is your responsibility and the responsibility of the state surveyors. We need to get those bad actors out. They need to be brought to justice, if you will. But for the most part, I just feel like I need to express to you the true quality work that many of these facilities provide and that many of these employees provide. And, Mr. Chairman, I will yield.

Mr. Harper. The gentleman yields back. The chair will now recognize the gentleman from Florida, Mr. Billirakis, for 5 minutes.

Mr. Bilirakis. Thank you, Mr. Chairman. I appreciate it. Thanks for holding this hearing, so very important.

As you know, Mr. Chairman, last year we had Irma that hit Florida. The many hardworking staff of our nursing homes and assisted living facilities prepared for the hurricane, 862 facilities evacuated, over 2,000 facilities lost power in the state of Florida. They were tested by the storm and the vast majority passed. Again those folks were doing the Lord's work and we do appreciate them so very much.

Yet, in every group there are bad actors as my colleague just said. We had the Rehabilitation Center at Hollywood Hills fail to take the proper measures to protect their residents and as a result 12 people died from heat exposure despite having a hospital across the street from the facility. These deaths were 100 percent preventable.

One of the concerns that have is how many facilities are not in compliance with the emergency rule. Dr. Goodrich, I believe that CMS began compliance surveys last year. That is my understanding. Do we know how many facilities are currently not in compliance with the emergency rule? That is my first question.

Dr. Goodrich. Certainly. So we are about 75 percent of the way through surveying all facilities nationally for the emergency preparedness requirements. We will have completed surveys for a hundred percent of facilities by February of 2019. While we are finding that the majority of facilities are in compliance or come into compliance quickly, we have had some citations for noncompliance that are intended to swiftly bring these facilities into compliance. So we have had about 2,300 facilities or so, so far, be cited for noncompliance that then would have to implement a corrective action plan in order to come into compliance.

Mr. Bilirakis. So 2,300 out of how many?

Dr. Goodrich. There's a total of about 15,600 nursing homes but again they haven't all been surveyed yet.

Mr. Bilirakis. Right, so but the majority of them have been surveyed.

Dr. Goodrich. Seventy five percent about.

Mr. Bilirakis. OK, thank you. The rehab center had their provider agreement terminated. This is the one that I was speaking of in Hollywood, Florida. It was terminated by CMS. Despite this, the owner of the rehab center still has an ownership stake in 11 other facilities that participate in the Medicare program. These facilities continue to operate despite the tragedy that occurred last year and the previous allegations that the Department of Justice made against the owner regarding providing unnecessary medical treatment to seniors.

Dr. Goodrich, given your experience at CMS, are you surprised by this that there are so many, he is operating so many other facilities? And yes and is he being monitored? Can you maybe expand on that, please?

Dr. Goodrich. Certainly. So for any Medicare-certified facility of any type they are required to undergo surveys just like nursing homes do, so whatever type of facility an owner may have an ownership interest in. So they have to undergo periodic recertification surveys in the situation of nursing homes, those are annual. And then there's complaint surveys that can take place if somebody files a quality of care complaint.

So any facility no matter what type that is Medicare-certified would have to undergo these surveys as well.

Mr. Bilirakis. OK, can you maybe get back to me on whether these other 12 facilities that this person owns follow the emergency rule? Can you give me that information? I know you can't, more than likely you don't have it with you now.

Dr. Goodrich. What I do know is that the other facilities owned by this owner have undergone the standard recertification surveys. As it relates specifically to emergency preparedness we will have to get back to you on that.

Mr. Bilirakis. Please get back to me on that. I appreciate it. Again, Doctor, I know the State is trying to pull the rehab center's owners licenses, but I am told it is tied up in the court system at the moment. I know I don't have a lot of time, so can CMS terminate the provider agreements with the various facilities that he has an ownership stake in? Do you have the ability to do that?

Dr. Goodrich. As I understand it, Medicare has the ability to bar an individual from owning other facilities under two circumstances. One is if they have a felony conviction and the second is if they're on the OIG exclusion list.

Mr. Bilirakis. OK, very good.

Well, thank you, Mr. Chairman. Thanks for allowing me to sit in and thanks for holding this hearing. I appreciate it.

Mr. Harper. The gentleman yields back.

Just a little quick follow-up to you, Ms. Dorrill, and to you, Mr. Dicken. Both HHS OIG and GAO have found situations where these allegations of abuse or neglect or substandard care they have been reported but state survey agencies failed to investigate those claims in a timely manner. CMS reserves immediate jeopardy classifications for situations that have caused or are likely to cause a serious injury, harm, or death to a resident and require such a claim to be investigated within 2 days.

So, Ms. Dorrill and Mr. Dicken, when state survey agencies fail to conduct those timely investigations especially in cases of immediate jeopardy, does that place nursing home residents at greater risk?

Mr. Dicken. Certainly as we've looked at the complaint investigation processes we've seen that States have sometimes been challenged to meet timeframes better at the immediate jeopardy types of issues that you raise. We did see, however, that as States are not timely it's much more difficult for States to be able to substantiate allegations and there are higher substantiation when they are meeting timely frameworks. So it is important to have a timely and complete complaint investigation.

Mr. Harper. All right. Well, let me follow up on that. So does this failure also potentially allow facilities which may have in fact harmed a resident to go unpunished and perhaps give a false impression that they are providing a better standard of care than they actually are?

Mr. Dicken. Well, certainly to the extent that the complaints are not investigated or not investigated in a timely manner that as you know can make it hard to substantiate. Certainly there are other processes that can go in and identify that as part of the standard survey process, but that is a real concern that if they are not being substantiated and because of not timely reviews.

Mr. Harper. Thank you.

Ms. Dorrill, anything you would like to add to that?

Ms. Dorrill. Just to reiterate how important timeliness is in terms of substantiation. We did find that there were only a handful of States who had substantial problems with that to the extent that that's helpful.

Mr. Harper. I want to thank each of you for being here. Our concern is the care and well-being of the residents of any of these facilities. They are the loved ones of many families that care greatly about what happens. You have a great responsibility. We thank you for being here today.

I also want to remind members that they have 10 business days to submit questions for the record, and should you receive any of those as witnesses from today we would appreciate your response as promptly as possible to that. With that the subcommittee is adjourned.

[Whereupon, at 12:00 p.m., the subcommittee was adjourned.] [Material submitted for inclusion in the record follows:]

E&C EST. 1795 U.S. HOUSE OF REPRESENTATIVES
COMMITTEE ON ENERGY AND COMMERCE

September 4, 2018

TO: Members, Subcommittee on Oversight and Investigations
FROM: Committee Majority Staff
RE: Hearing entitled "Examining Federal Efforts to Ensure Quality of Care and Resident Safety in Nursing Homes."

The Subcommittee on Oversight and Investigations will hold a hearing on Thursday, September 6, 2018, at 10:15 a.m. in 2322 Rayburn House Office Building, entitled "Examining Federal Efforts to Ensure Quality of Care and Resident Safety in Nursing Homes." The purpose of the hearing is to explore the roles of the Centers for Medicare and Medicaid Services (CMS) and the Office of Inspector General at the U.S. Department of Health and Human Services (HHS OIG) relating to the management and safety of nursing home facilities.

Witnesses

- Kate Goodrich, M.D., Director, Center for Clinical Standards and Quality, and Chief Medical Officer, CMS;
- Ruth Ann Dorrill, Regional Inspector General, HHS OIG; and
- John Dicken, Director, Health Care, Government Accountability Office (GAO).

Background

The Committee on Energy and Commerce (the Committee) began conducting oversight of nursing homes after numerous media reports described instances of abuse, neglect, and substandard care occurring at SNFs and NFs across the country, including the Rehabilitation Center at Hollywood Hills where at least 12 residents died in the immediate aftermath of Hurricane Irma in September 2017.[47]

---

[47] *See, e.g.*, NH Staff, *Nursing home lawyers a no-show in records case*, NAPLES HERALD, May 22, 2018, http://naplesherald.com/2018/05/22/nursing-home-lawyers-a-no-show-in-records-

Management Failure at the Rehabilitation Center at Hollywood Hills

On October 20, 2017, the Committee sent a bipartisan letter requesting documents and information from Jack Michel, an owner of the Rehabilitation Center at Hollywood Hills (Rehabilitation Center) where at least 12 residents died in the immediate aftermath of Hurricane Irma in Florida.[48] The Committee raised concerns about the organization's failure to protect the health, safety, and welfare of residents at the facility.[49] According to the Florida Agency for Health Care Administration (AHCA), the Rehabilitation Center failed to follow adequate emergency management procedures after the facility's air conditioning system lost power during Hurricane Irma.[50] Despite increasingly excessive heat, staff at the facility did not take advantage of a fully functional hospital across the street and "overwhelmingly delayed calling 911" during a medical emergency.[51]

The facility also had contractual agreements with an assisted living facility and transportation company for emergency evacuation purposes yet did not activate these services.[52] CMS ultimately terminated the Rehabilitation Center from the Medicare and Medicaid programs following an on-site inspection where surveyors found that the facility failed to meet

---

case/; Blake Ellis and Melanie Hicken, *Sick, Dying and Raped in America's Nursing Homes*, CNN, Feb. 22, 2017, http://www.cnn.com/interactive/2017/02/health/nursing-home-sex-abuse-investigation/.

[48] Letter from Hon. Greg Walden, Chairman, H. Comm. on Energy & Commerce, et al., to Dr. Jack Michel, Owner, Rehabilitation Center at Hollywood Hills, LLC (Oct. 20, 2017), *available at* https://energycommerce.house.gov/wp-content/uploads/2017/10/20171020HollywoodHills.pdf; *See also* NH Staff, *supra* note 1.

[49] Letter from Hon. Greg Walden, Chairman, H. Comm. on Energy & Commerce, et al., to Dr. Jack Michel, Owner, Rehabilitation Center at Hollywood Hills, LLC (Oct. 20, 2017).

[50] Florida Agency for Health Care Administration, *Press Release: AHCA Suspends the License of the Rehabilitation Center of Hollywood Hills* (Sept. 20, 2017); Paul McMahon, et al., *Ninth nursing home patient dies; Gov. Scott details contact with state*, SUN SENTINEL, Sept. 19, 2018, http://www.sun-sentinel.com/news/hollywood-nursing-home-hurricane-deaths/fl-reg-nursing-home-ninth-death-20170919-story.html.

[51] AHCA Press Release, *ACHA Suspends the License of the Rehabilitation Center of Hollywood Hills*, (Sept. 20, 2017); U.S. Dep't of Health and Human Services, Centers for Medicare and Medicaid Services (CMS), Survey of the Rehabilitation Center at Hollywood Hills, LLC, at 2 (Sept. 22, 2017); *State of Florida, Agency for Health Care Administration vs. Rehabilitation Center at Hollywood Hills, LLC*, Emergency Suspension Order (Sept. 20, 2017).

[52] U.S. Dep't of Health and Human Services, Centers for Medicare and Medicaid Services (CMS), Survey of the Rehabilitation Center at Hollywood Hills, LLC (Sept. 22, 2017).

Medicare's basic health and safety requirements.[53] During a hearing before the Subcommittee on Oversight and Investigations in October 2017, CMS described the events at this nursing home as a "complete management failure."[54]

On November 17, 2017, Dr. Michel provided a response through his attorney to the Committee's inquiry, contending among other things, that the facility made patients as comfortable as possible during the loss of air conditioning.[55] According to the letter, "although AC power was lost on September 10, Hollywood Hills continued to otherwise have electrical power, and deployed eight 'spot coolers' (portable air conditioning units that had been purchased as part of hurricane preparedness) and numerous fans through the building in an effort to keep residents as comfortable as possible, given the loss of central air conditioning."[56] However, according to an engineer testifying in the ongoing litigation between the Rehabilitation Center and the State of Florida, Hollywood Hills failed to properly ventilate the portable coolers which resulted in increased temperatures in most of the facility, particularly the second floor where the majority of deaths occurred.[57] According to the expert, the coolers operated by the facility "made it worse."[58]

---

[53] U.S. Dep't of Health and Human Services, Centers for Medicare and Medicaid Services, *Notice to Public of Rehabilitation Center at Hollywood Hills, Termination Notice* (Oct. 11, 2017), *available at* https://www.cms.gov/Medicare/Provider-Enrollment-and-Certification/SurveyCertificationGenInfo/Downloads/ Termination-Notice-Florida-NH-Rehabilitation-Center-at-Hollywood-Hills-LLC.pdf.

[54] *Examining HHS's Public Health Preparedness for and Response to the 2017 Hurricane Season: Hearing Before the Subcomm. On Oversight & Investigations of the H. Comm. On Energy and Commerce*, 115th Cong., Preliminary Transcript, 108 (Oct. 24, 2017) *available at* https://docs.house.gov/meetings/IF/IF02/20171024/106530/HHRG-115- IF02-Transcript-20171024.pdf.

[55] Letter from Geoffrey D. Smith, Atty., Smith & Associates, to Hon. Greg Walden, Chairman, H. Comm. on Energy & Commerce, et al., (Nov. 17, 2017) (On file with the Committee).

[56] *Id.*

[57] Deposition of William Scott Crawford, PE, *State of FL for Healthcare Admin. Vs. Rehabilitation Center at Hollywood Hills*, Feb. 16, 2018, available at; *see also* Terry Spencer, *Expert: Coolers Made it Worse in Nursing Home Where 12 Died*, ASSOCIATED PRESS, Mar. 23, 2018, https://www.yahoo.com/news/expert-coolers-made- worse-nursing-home-where-12-185954138.html; Erika Pesantes, et. al, *Second Floor was Deadliest at Nursing Home with No Air Conditioning*, SUN SENTINEL, Oct. 6, 2017, http://www.sun-sentinel.com/news/hollywood-nursing-home-hurricane-deaths/fl-sb-nursing-home-sunrise-hollywood-20170927-story.html.

[58] *Id.*

Past Allegations Involving Dr. Michel and Corporate Integrity Agreement

The Committee's investigation and public reports revealed that facilities affiliated with Dr. Michel have been the subject of federal government scrutiny for over a decade. In 2006, Larkin Community Hospital (Larkin), and others entered into a settlement agreement with the Department of Justice (DOJ) to resolve a civil case in which the government alleged Dr. Michel and his associates paid kickbacks and performed medically unnecessary treatments on elderly beneficiaries to generate Medicare and Medicaid payments.[59] According to DOJ's complaint, Dr. Michel initiated the scheme during a meeting with an associate of the then-owner of a nearby hospital, Larkin by proposing, "ask your boss if he would pay $1 million to make $5 million."[60] Thereafter, Dr. Michel and his associates allegedly entered into a scheme to engage in seven different types of kickback arrangements.[61]

Dr. Michel and the parties eventually settled with DOJ for $15.4 million without an admission of guilt.[62] With the settlement, Larkin and Dr. Michel entered into a five-year Corporate Integrity Agreement (CIA) with HHS OIG in 2006.[63] Despite the CIA, media reports indicate that from approximately 2002 to 2016, at least one then-employee and physicians at

---

[59] U.S. Dep't of Justice, Press Release, *Miami Hospital Pays $15.4 Million to Resolve Fraud Case for Kickbacks & Medically Unnecessary Treatments* (Nov. 30, 2006), *available at* https://www.justice.gov/archive/opa/pr/2006/November/06_civ_803.html.

[60] *United States v. Jack Jacob Michel, et al.*, Complaint of the United States, No-04-21579-CIV-JORDAN/TORRES, at 31 (Filed Jun. 29, 2004) (S.D. Fla.).

[61] *Id.* at 30-36.

[62] U.S. Dep't of Justice, Press Release, *Miami Hospital Pays $15.4 Million to Resolve Fraud Case for Kickbacks & Medically Unnecessary Treatments* (Nov. 30, 2006) *available at* https://www.justice.gov/archive/opa/pr/2006/November/06_civ_803.html; *See also United States v. Philip Esformes*, Government's Motion for Pre-Trial Detention and Supporting Memorandum, Case No. 16-20549, at Attachment B, Page 6 (Filed Jul. 22, 2016) (S.D. Fla.) (Attachment B includes Settlement Agreement Binder from *United States v. Michel* ("Civil Action"), No-04-21579-CIV-JORDAN/TORRES (S.D. Fla.)).

[63] U.S. Dep't of Health and Human Services, Office of Inspector General, Integrity Agreement Between the Office of Inspector General of the Dep't of Health and Human Services and Jack J. Michel, M.D. (Nov. 17, 2006); U.S. Dep't of Health and Human Services, Office of Inspector General, Integrity Agreement Between the Office of Inspector General of the Dep't of Health and Human Services and Larkin Community Hospital (Nov. 13, 2006).

Larkin were allegedly involved in the largest single criminal health care fraud case ever brought against individuals by DOJ.[64]

Dr. Michel Continues to Own Multiple Health Care Related Facilities Participating in Federal Programs

Last year, state regulators in Florida raised concerns about patient safety at another facility owned by Dr. Michel.[65] In December 2016, the AHCA found 30 violations at Floridian Gardens Assisted Living Facility, including "sexual assault of patients, low staffing, and ignoring patients."[66] As a result, the facility was banned from accepting new patients for several months.[67] In September 2017, the AHCA took additional steps to close Floridian Gardens.[68] According to information obtained by the Committee from CMS, Dr. Michel currently has an ownership interest in at least 11 health care related facilities enrolled in Medicare despite the tragedy at the Rehabilitation Center and other previous instances of apparent wrongdoing.[69]

Emergency Preparedness at SNFs and NFs

Emergency preparedness is a critical issue for long-term care facilities, and CMS requires that Medicare- and Medicaid-certified nursing homes comply with certain federal requirements regarding emergency preparedness. HHS OIG has examined some of these requirements, issuing reports in 2006 and 2012 regarding emergency preparedness and response

---

[64] Jay Weaver, *Bribes to low-paid state worker key to $1 billion Miami Medicare fraud case, prosecutors say*, MIAMI HERALD, Jul. 29, 2017, http://www.miamiherald.com/news/local/article164232522.html; *See also* U.S. Dep't of Justice, Press Release, *Three Individuals Charged in $1 Billion Medicare Fraud and Money Laundering Scheme* (Jul. 22, 2016), *available at* https://www.justice.gov/opa/pr/three-individuals-charged-1-billion-medicare-fraud-and- money-laundering-scheme.

[65] Melanie Payne & Arek Sarkissian, *Nursing Home Deaths: Owner's Other Facility Faced State Ban on New Patients*, USA TODAY NETWORK FLORIDA, Sept. 15, 2017, https://www.usatoday.com/story/news/nation-now/2017/09/15/nursing-home-deaths-owners-other-facility-faced-state-ban-new-patients/672340001/.

[66] *Id.*

[67] *Id.*

[68] *See* Florida Agency for Health Care Administration, *Press Release: AHCA Takes Additional Action to Close Larkin-Owned ALF* (Sept. 28, 2017), https://www.ahca.myflorida.com/Executive/Communications/Press_Releases/pdf/Larkin-OwnedALFPR.pdf.

[69] E-mail from Staff, Centers for Medicare and Medicaid Services to Staff, H. Comm. on Energy & Commerce (May 11, 2018. 5:12 pm) (On file with the Committee).

in nursing homes.[70] In these reports, HHS OIG found that there were gaps in nursing home preparedness and response and made recommendations to CMS to update and revise certain federal requirements regarding emergency preparedness.[71]

Over the past decade, CMS has adopted new policies and procedures to improve emergency preparedness in nursing homes and other health care facilities. For example, in 2007, CMS issued three emergency preparedness checklists for health care facilities (including nursing homes), State Long Term Care (LTC) Ombudsman programs, and State Survey Agencies.[72] More recently, in September 2016, CMS finalized a new emergency preparedness rule for Medicare and Medicaid participating providers and suppliers that imposed new requirements on 17 different provides/suppliers, including long-term care facilities.[73] The rule, among other things, outlined four core elements of the Emergency Preparedness Program for all provider types (*i.e.*, Risk Assessment and Planning, Policies and Procedures, Communication Plan, and Training and Testing).[74] At the Subcommittee's October 2017 hearing entitled "Examining HHS's Public Health Preparedness for and Response to the 2017 Hurricane Season," CMS was asked about its emergency preparedness requirements and testified that the surveyors would begin surveying for the new rule starting in November 2017 and that the rule required, among other things, generators, emergency preparedness plans, and training on a continual basis.[75]

---

[70] U.S. Dep't of Health and Human Services, Office of the Inspector General, *Nursing Home Emergency Preparedness and Response During Recent Hurricanes*, OEI-06-06-00020 (Aug. 2006) *available at* https://oig.hhs.gov/oei/reports/oei-06-06-00020.pdf; U.S. Dep't of Health and Human Services, Office of Inspector General, *Gaps Continue to Exist in Nursing Home Emergency Preparedness and Response During Disasters: 2007-2010*, OEI-06-09-00270 (Apr. 2012) *available at* https://oig.hhs.gov/oei/reports/oei-06-09-00270.pdf.

[71] *Id.*

[72] U.S. Dep't of Health and Human Services, Office of Inspector General, *Gaps Continue to Exist in Nursing Home Emergency Preparedness and Response During Disasters: 2007-2010*, OEI-06-09-00270, at 5 (Apr. 2012).

[73] Centers for Medicare and Medicaid Services, *Emergency Preparedness Rule*, CMS.GOV (last updated Jul. 9, 2018), *available at* https://www.cms.gov/Medicare/Provider-Enrollment-and- Certification/SurveyCertEmergPrep/Emergency-Prep-Rule.html.

[74] *Id.*

[75] The compliance deadline for the new rule was November 15, 2017. *Id.*; *Examining HHS's Public Health Preparedness for and Response to the 2017 Hurricane Season: Hearing*

CMS Oversight of National Nursing Homes

On April 2, 2018, the Committee wrote to CMS Administrator Seema Verma, requesting documents and information relating to CMS' oversight of SNFs and NFs participating in the Medicare and Medicaid programs.[76] Media reports cited in the letter described instances of nursing home residents being abused and neglected and, in some instances, the nursing homes subsequently failing to detect and investigate adequately the abuse and neglect.[77] Analysis conducted by one news outlet found that between 2013 and 2016, the federal government cited more than 1,000 nursing homes for either mishandling cases related to, or failing to protect residents against, rape, sexual abuse, or sexual assault, with nearly 100 facilities incurring multiple citations.[78] The Centers for Disease Control (CDC) National Center for Health Statistics found that, as of 2014, there were 15,600 nursing home facilities in the United States; 69.8 percent of U.S. nursing home facilities have for-profit ownership.[79]

For over a decade, HHS OIG has identified improving care for vulnerable populations, including the care provided to individuals receiving nursing home care, as a top management challenge for HHS and has continuously expressed concerns about residents being at risk of abuse and neglect.[80] According to HHS OIG's 2017 report on top management challenges:

Before the Subcomm. On Oversight & Investigations of the H. Comm. On Energy and Commerce, 115th Cong., Preliminary Transcript, 108 (Oct. 24, 2017) *available at* https://docs.house.gov/meetings/IF/IF02/20171024/106530/HHRG-115-IF02-Transcript-20171024.pdf.

[76] Letter from Hon. Greg Walden, Chairman, H. Comm. on Energy & Commerce, et al., to Hon. Seema Verma, Administrator, Centers for Medicare & Medicaid Services (Nov. 17, 2017) *available at* https://energycommerce.house.gov/wp-content/uploads/2018/04/20180402CMS.pdf.

[77] Ellis and Hicken, *supra* note 1.

[78] *Id.*

[79] Centers for Disease Control and Prevention, *Nursing Home Care* (last updated May 3, 2017) *available at* https://www.cdc.gov/nchs/fastats/nursing-home-care.htm.

[80] U.S. Dep't of Health and Human Services, Office of Inspector General, *Top Management and Performance Challenges Facing HHS 2017, #4 Improving Care for Vulnerable Populations* (last accessed Aug. 29, 2018), https://oig.hhs.gov/reports-and-publications/top-challenges/2017/2017-tmc.pdf; U.S. Dep't of Health and Human Services, Office of Inspector General, *Top Management and Performance Challenges Facing HHS 2016, #7 Ensuring Quality of Care and Safety for Vulnerable Populations* (last accessed Aug. 29, 2018), https://oig.hhs.gov/reports-and-publications/top-

> Nursing facilities continue to experience problems ensuring quality of care and safety for people residing in them. OIG identified instances of substandard care causing preventable adverse events, finding an estimated 22 percent of Medicare beneficiaries had experienced an adverse event during their nursing stay.[81]

The report further states that "OIG continues to raise concerns about nursing home residents being at risk of abuse and neglect. In some instances, nursing home care is so substandard that providers may have liability under the False Claims Act."[82]

In addition, GAO has developed a substantial body of work wherein CMS' efforts to ensure that nursing home residents are free from abuse and receive the proper standard of care have been called into question.[83]

Oversight of Nursing Homes: Surveys, Deficiencies, and Corrective Action Plans

HHS utilizes state health agencies or other state agencies to determine if nursing homes meet the minimum federal requirements for participation

---

hallenges/2016/TMC_2016_508.pdf; U.S. Dep't of Health and Human Services, Office of Inspector General, *OIG's FY 2015 Top Management and Performance Challenges Facing the Department of Health and Human Services, Management Challenge 6: Ensuring Quality in Nursing Home, Hospice, and Home- and Community-Based Care* (last accessed Aug. 29, 2018), https://oig.hhs.gov/reports- and-publications/top-challenges/2015/2015-tmc.pdf.

[81] 2017 Management Challenges, *supra* note 34.

[82] *Id.*

[83] *See* U.S. GOV'T ACCOUNTABILITY OFFICE, GAO-16-33, Nursing Home Quality: CMS Should Continue to Improve Data and Oversight (2015) *available at* https://www.gao.gov/assets/680/673480.pdf. *See also* U.S. GOV'T ACCOUNTABILITY OFFICE, GAO-11-280, Nursing Homes: More Reliable Data and Consistent Guidance Would Improve CMS Oversight of State Complaint Investigations (2011) *available at* https://www.gao.gov/assets/320/317514.pdf; U.S. GOV'T ACCOUNTABILITY OFFICE, GAO-10-197, Poorly Performing Nursing Homes: Special Focus Facilities Are Often Improving, but CMS's Program Could be Strengthened (2010) *available at* https://www.gao.gov/assets/310/302117.pdf; U.S. GOV'T ACCOUNTABILITY OFFICE, GAO-10-70, Nursing Homes: Addressing the Factors Underlying Understatement of Serious Care Problems Requires Sustained CMS and State Commitment (2009) *available at* https://www.gao.gov/assets/300/298953.pdf; U.S. GOV'T ACCOUNTABILITY OFFICE, GAO-08-517, Nursing Homes: Federal Monitoring Surveys Demonstrate Continued Understatement of Serious Care Problems and CMS Oversight Weaknesses (2008) *available at* https://www.gao.gov/assets/280/275154.pdf; and U.S. GOV'T ACCOUNTABILITY OFFICE, GAO-07-241, Nursing Homes: Efforts to Strengthen Federal Enforcement Have Not Deterred Some Homes for Repeatedly Harming Residents (2007) *available at* https://www.gao.gov/assets/260/258016.pdf.

in the Medicare and Medicaid programs (hereinafter "Conditions of Participation" or "CoPs").[84] Accordingly, through an agreement with HHS, the state agency is required to "conduct standard surveys to determine whether nursing homes are in compliance with Federal participation requirements."[85] A standard survey is defined as "a periodic nursing home inspection," using procedures specified in CMS' *State Operations Manual* (hereinafter "Manual"), "that focuses on a sample of residents selected by the state agency to gather information about the quality of resident care furnished to Medicare or Medicaid beneficiaries in a nursing home."[86] A survey must take place at each facility "at least once every 15 months."[87] However, each state must maintain a statewide average of conducting surveys once every 12 months.[88] Nursing homes that do not achieve substantial compliance within six months will be terminated from participating in Medicare and Medicaid.[89]

The state is also required to review "complaint allegations" with the option to "conduct a standard survey or an abbreviated standard (complaint survey) to investigate noncompliance with the CoPs.[90] "A nursing home's noncompliance with a Federal participation requirement is defined as a deficiency."[91] The state agency determines the deficiency rating utilizing severity and scope components.[92] Each deficiency is assigned a letter rating of A to L, with L being the most serious and A the least.[93]

Severity is the degree of or potential for resident harm and has four levels, beginning with the most severe: (1) immediate jeopardy to resident health or safety, (2) actual harm that is not immediate jeopardy, (3) no

---

[84] *See* U.S. Dep't of Health and Human Services, *Office of Inspector General, Kansas Did Not Always Verify Correction of Deficiencies Identified During Surveys of Nursing Homes Participating in Medicare and Medicaid* (A-07-17-03218), Sept. 2017, *available at* https://oig.hhs.gov/oas/reports/region7/71703218.pdf.

[85] *Id.*

[86] *Id.*

[87] *Id.*

[88] 42 U.S.C. § 1395i–3(g)(2)(A)(iii)(I) and 42 U.S.C. § 1396r (g)(2)(A)(iii)(I).

[89] CMS Nursing Home Enforcement, *available at* https://www.cms.gov/Medicare/Provider-Enrollment-and-Certification/SurveyCertificationEnforcement/Nursing-Home-Enforcement.html. *See also* 42 U.S.C. § 1395i-3(h)(2)(C) and 42 U.S.C. § 1396r(h)(3)(D).

[90] HHS OIG Report, *supra* note 38.

[91] *Id.*

[92] *Id.*

[93] *Id.*

actual harm with potential for more than minimal harm but not immediate jeopardy, and (4) no actual harm with potential for minimal harm. Scope is the number of residents affected or pervasiveness of the deficiency in the nursing home and has three levels: (1) isolated, (2) pattern, (3) widespread. The Manual provides information on the severity and scope of levels used to determine the deficiency rating.[94]

Table 2. Severity and Scope Levels for Deficiency Ratings[95]

	Scope		
Severity	**Isolated**	**Pattern**	**Widespread**
Immediate jeopardy to resident health or safety	J	K	L
Actual harm that is not immediate jeopardy	G	H	I
No actual harm with potential for more than minimal harm but not immediate jeopardy	D	E	F
No actual harm with potential for minimal harm	A	B	C

Nursing homes are required to submit corrective actions plans to either the appropriate state agency or CMS, detailing how the nursing home corrected the deficiency or plans to correct the deficiency.[96] After receiving the plan, the state or CMS certifies whether the facility is in substantial compliance with the CoPs.[97] Substantial compliance occurs when "there is substantial compliance by verifying correction of the identified deficiencies through obtaining evidence of correction or conducting an onsite review."[98]

According to information provided to the Committee by CMS, the number of complaint surveys with deficiencies cited at the immediate

---

[94] *Id.*

[95] U.S. Dep't of Health and Human Services, Office of Inspector General, *Florida Did Not Always Verify Correction of Deficiencies Identified During Surveys of Nursing Homes Participating in Medicare and Medicaid*, A-04-17-0852 (Apr. 2018) *available at* https://oig.hhs.gov/oas/reports/region4/41708052.pdf.

[96] HHS OIG Report, *supra* note 38.

[97] *Id.*

[98] *Id.*

jeopardy level has increased each of the last four years. In 2013, there were 1,250 complaints at the immediate jeopardy level compared to 1,801 in 2017, the most recent data available—an increase of more than 44 percent.[99]

Delays Reviewing Complaint Allegations

While staffing shortages continue to be an issue for a variety of reasons in the nursing home industry and at state agencies, some nursing home residents appear to be placed in unsafe situations because of a lack of oversight by state agencies and CMS.[100] A September 2017 Data Brief issued by the HHS OIG found that in 2015, 764 immediate jeopardy nursing home complaints were not investigated by state agencies within two working days, as required by CMS, and 473 complaints were not investigated within 15 days.[101] Immediate jeopardy is described by CMS as being instances where "the facility's noncompliance with more or more requirements of participation has caused, or is likely to cause, serious injury, harm, impairment, or death to a resident."[102] HHS OIG also found that 4,743 high priority nursing home complaints were not investigated in 2015 within the required 10 working day period.[103]

However, it should also be noted that failing to properly address and administer complaint investigations has been a long-standing problem for state agencies and CMS. For example, a report issued by the U.S. General

---

[99] Centers for Medicare and Medicaid Services, *supra* note 23. Federal law requires states to maintain procedures and adequate staff to investigate complaints of violations of federal requirements by SNFs and NFs. *See* 42 U.S.C. § 1395i-3(g)(4)(A) and 42 U.S.C. § 1396r(g)(4)(A).

[100] *See* John Caniglia & Jo Ellen Corrigan, *Ohio Nursing Home Inspectors Fail to Meet Federal Deadlines Amid Serious Understaffing: A Critical Choice*, THE PLAIN DEALER, Apr 23, 2017, *available at* https://www.cleveland.com/metro/index.ssf/2017/04/ohio_nursing_home_inspectors_f.html.i

[101] U.S. Dep't of Health and Human Services, Office of Inspector General, *A Few States Fell Short in Timely Investigation of the Most Serious Nursing Home Complaints: 2011-2015* (OEI-01-16-00330) (Sept. 2017) *available at* https://oig.hhs.gov/oei/reports/oei-01-16-00330.pdf.

[102] *Id.*

[103] *Id.*

Accounting Office[104] in 1999 found that "[s]erious complaints alleging that nursing home residents are being harmed can remain uninvestigated for weeks or months. Such delays can prolong situations in which residents may be subject to abuse, neglect resulting in serious care problems like malnutrition and dehydration, preventable accidents, and medication errors."[105] According to the report, CMS (then known as the Health Care Financing Administration (HCFA))[106] had only established minimal standards for complaint investigations and did not perform adequate oversight to ensure resident complaints were being investigated in a timely manner.[107] HHS OIG also made similar findings in a 2006 report, once again noting inadequacies in CMS' oversight.[108]

Correction of Deficiencies Not Always Verified

HHS OIG has also issued several reports examining whether states always verified correction of deficiencies identified during surveys of nursing homes participating in Medicare and Medicaid.[109] While in some instances HHS OIG found that states properly verified correction of deficiencies identified during surveys of nursing homes,[110] HHS OIG

---

104 The U.S. General Accounting Office was renamed the U.S. Government Accountability Office (GAO) in July 2004. *See* GAO Human Capital Reform Act of 2004, Pub. L. 108-271, 118 Stat. 811 (2004).

105 U.S. GEN. ACCOUNTING OFFICE, GAO/HEHS-99-80, Nursing Homes: Complaint Investigation Process Often Inadequate to Protect Residents (1999) *available at* https://www.gao.gov/assets/230/227108.pdf.

106 CNN, *Medicare agency renamed as prelude to reforms*, CNN, June 14, 2001, http://www.cnn.com/2001/HEALTH/06/14/hcfa.changes/.

107 U.S. GEN. ACCOUNTING OFFICE, *supra* note 59.

108 U.S. Dep't of Health and Human Services, Office of Inspector General, *Nursing Home Complaint Investigations* (OEI-01-04-00340) (July 2006) *available at* https://oig.hhs.gov/oei/reports/oei-01-04-00340.pdf.

109 According to a May 2018 report issued by HHS OIG, OIG had released 15 reports related to this topic. *See, e.g.,* U.S. Dep't of Health and Human Services, Office of Inspector General, *Nebraska Did Not Always Verify Correction of Deficiencies Identified During Surveys of Nursing Homes Participating in Medicare and Medicaid*, A-07-17-03224 (May 2018) *available at* https://oig.hhs.gov/oas/reports/region7/71703224.pdf.

110 *See, e.g.*, U.S. Dep't of Health and Human Services, Office of Inspector General, *Missouri Properly Verified Correction of Deficiencies Identified During Surveys of Nursing Homes*, A-07-16-03217 (Mar. 17, 2017) *available at* https://oig.hhs.gov/oas/reports/region7/71603217.pdf; U.S. Dep't of Health and Human Services, Office of Inspector General, *Oregon Properly Verified Correction of Deficiencies Identified During Surveys of Nursing Homes Participating in Medicare and Medicaid*, A-

generally found that states did not always verify correction of deficiencies identified during surveys of nursing homes participating in Medicare and Medicaid.[111] For example, in September 2017, HHS OIG released a report finding that Kansas did not always verify whether nursing homes corrected deficiencies.[112] The report found that, out of 100 sampled deficiencies identified during CY 2014 surveys, Kansas failed to adequately verify that the deficiencies were corrected 52 percent of the time.[113] HHS OIG also found that the state failed to conduct required standard surveys within the required 15-month timeframe for 35 of 79 nursing homes in CY 2014.[114] According to a recent media report, Kansas "may conduct less than 40% of required nursing home surveys" during 2018.[115]

Inconsistency of Penalties

According to information reviewed by the Committee, there appears to be variation in penalties among states and regions relating to how civil monetary penalties (CMPs) are assessed. In some cases, there is little to no correlation between the severity of deficiency and the resulting civil monetary penalty. Even within the same state, some facilities can incur significant civil monetary penalties despite not having any serious deficiencies while other facilities may have been cited for several deficiencies yet incur little to no penalties. For example, at least one nursing home did not incur any financial penalty even after being cited for not protecting residents after a case of sexual abuse was sustained.[116] There also appears to be a variation relating to intra-facility penalties. For instance, some facilities are cited for having serious deficiencies,

---

09-16-02007 (Mar. 14, 2016) *available at* https://oig.hhs.gov/oas/reports/region9/91602007.pdf.

[111] HHS OIG Report, *supra* note 63 at Appendix B.

[112] U.S. Dep't of Health and Human Services, Office of Inspector General, *Kansas Did Not Always Verify Correction of Deficiencies Identified During Surveys of Nursing Homes Participating in Medicare and Medicaid,* A-07-17-03218 (Sept. 2017) *available at* https://oig.hhs.gov/oas/reports/region7/71703218.pdf.

[113] *Id.*

[114] *Id.*

[115] Kimberly Marselas, MCKNIGHT'S LONG-TERM CARE NEWS, Apr. 26, 2018, https://www.mcknights.com/news/agency-may-conduct-less-than-40-of-required-nursing-home-surveys-in-kansas-this-year/article/761192/.

[116] Ellis and Hicken, *supra* note 1.

sometimes in successive surveys, yet incur little to no monetary penalties. Alternatively, these facilities may incur significant civil monetary penalties for deficiencies that are relatively low on CMS' severity scale.

1150B Authority Delegation

According to an August 2017 Early Alert, HHS OIG identified 134 Medicare beneficiaries who were treated in 2015 and 2016 for injuries that may have been caused by abuse or neglect when the individual was receiving care at a SNF.[117] HHS OIG raised concerns that CMS has inadequate procedures to ensure that incidents of potential abuse or neglect at SNFs are identified and reported in accordance with applicable requirements.[118] Under Section 1150B of the Social Security Act, covered individuals in federally funded SNFs and NFs are required to immediately report any reasonable suspicion of a crime committed against a resident of that facility.[119] The law imposes various penalties, including CMPs of up to $300,000 and possible exclusion from participation in federal health care programs, for failure to report possible crimes against SNF and NF residents.[120]

According to HHS OIG, CMS has not, however, taken any enforcement actions using section 1150B of the Social Security Act or used the penalties it contains despite its effective date of March 23, 2011.[121] CMS officials told HHS OIG that CMS has not taken any enforcement actions under 1150B "because the HHS Office of the Secretary has not delegated the enforcement of section 1150B to CMS[,]" and that it had "not identified any instances in which a covered individual failed to report an incident of potential abuse or neglect of a Medicare beneficiary."[122] CMS further indicated that it had commenced working

---

[117] U.S. Dep't of Health and Human Services, Office of Inspector General, *Early Alert: The Centers for Medicare & Medicaid Services Has Inadequate Procedures to Ensure That Incidents of Potential Abuse or Neglect at Skilled Nursing Facilities Are Identified and Reported in Accordance with Applicable Requirements* (A-01-17-00504) (Aug. 24, 2017) *available at* https://oig.hhs.gov/oas/reports/region1/11700504.pdf.

[118] *Id.*

[119] 42 U.S.C. § 1320b-25(b).

[120] 42 U.S.C. § 1320b-25(c).

[121] HHS OIG, *supra* note 71.

[122] *Id.*

with the HHS Office of the Secretary in June 2017 to obtain the delegated enforcement authority.[123] CMS is continuing to work on the delegation authority.

CMS' Administration of the Special Focus Facility (SFF) Program

As part of the Nursing Home Oversight and Improvement Program, the HCFA[124] created a Special Focus Facility (SFF) initiative in 1998.[125] The SFF program is designed to address nursing homes that have more problems than other nursing homes, more serious problems than most other nursing homes, and a pattern of serious problems that has persisted over a long period of time.[126] A facility is placed in the SFF program if the State Survey Agency selects the facility from a list of program candidates that is created by CMS.[127] As a SFF, the nursing home is subject to twice as many in-person visits by survey teams as other nursing homes and may face progressive enforcement actions.[128] CMS expects that within about 18-24 months the nursing home will: (1) improve and graduate from the SFF program; (2) be terminated from the Medicare and Medicaid programs; or (3) be provided with an extension of time to continue participating in the SFF program because the nursing home has made "very promising progress."[129]

---

[123] *Id.*

[124] The HCFA was renamed the Centers for Medicare & Medicaid Services (CMS) in June 2001. *See* CNN, *supra* note 60.

[125] *See* Statement of Alice Bonner, PhD, RN, Director of the Division of Nursing Homes, Office of Clinical Standards and Quality, Centers for Medicare & Medicaid Services Before the United States Senate Special Committee on Aging (July 2, 2012), *available at* https://www.aging.senate.gov/imo/media/doc/hr248ab.pdf.

[126] Centers for Medicare and Medicaid Services (CMS), *Special Focus Facility ("SFF") Initiative* (last updated Aug. 16, 2018), *available at* https://www.cms.gov/Medicare/Provider-Enrollment-and-Certification/CertificationandComplianc/NHs.html.

[127] *See* Centers for Medicare and Medicaid Services, *Center for Clinical Standards and Quality/Survey & Certification Group, Fiscal Year (FY) 2017 Special Focus Facility (SFF) Program Update* (Mar. 2, 2017), *available at* https://www.cms.gov/Medicare/Provider-Enrollment-and- Certification/SurveyCertificationGenInfo/Downloads/Survey-and-Cert-Letter-17-20.pdf.

[128] Centers for Medicare and Medicaid Services (CMS), *Special Focus Facility ("SFF") Initiative* (last updated Aug. 16, 2018), *available at* https://www.cms.gov/Medicare/Provider-Enrollment-and-Certification/CertificationandComplianc/NHs.html.

[129] *Id.*

Since the program's creation, CMS has made improvements to the program to, among other things, increase the number of nursing homes participating in the program, strengthen enforcement, enhance transparency, and rate all nursing homes using a Five-Star Quality Rating System.[130] As of August 16, 2018, there were a total of 85 facilities in the SFF program, including 20 newly added facilities to the SFF program, 33 facilities in the SFF program that had not improved, 32 facilities in the SFF program that had shown improvement, and 25 facilities that had recently graduated from the SFF program.[131] According to CMS' August 16, 2018 update regarding facilities in the SFF program, the amount of time that the current facilities in the SFF program have been in the program ranges from 0 months to 47 months.[132] Some of these facilities have been in the program longer than CMS' expected 24 months, as the list shows that two facilities have been in the SFF program for more than 24 months and have not improved and 4 facilities have been in the SFF for more than 24 months and have shown improvement.[133]

It is important to note that the SFF program does not supersede the statutory requirement that a nursing home be terminated from the Medicare and/or Medicaid program if it does not achieve substantial compliance with federal requirements within six months of the date of the first findings of noncompliance.[134]

Updated SNF and NF Conditions of Participation

Congress enacted the Federal Nursing Home Reform Act (hereinafter "Act" or "Nursing Home Reform Act") as part of the Omnibus Budget Reconciliation Act of 1987.[135] The enactment of the Nursing Home Reform Act followed the publication of a comprehensive study conducted by the

---

130 Centers for Medicare and Medicaid Services (CMS), *Special Focus Facility ("SFF") Initiative* (last updated Aug. 16, 2018), *available at* https://www.cms.gov/Medicare/Provider-Enrollment-and- Certification/CertificationandComplianc/NHs.html.

131 *Id.*

132 *Id.*

133 *Id.*

134 *See* CMS, *supra* note 81. *See also* 42 U.S.C. § 1395i-3(h)(2)(C) and 42 U.S.C. § 1396r(h)(3)(D).

135 Omnibus Budget Reconciliation Act of 1987, Pub. L. No. 100-203, 101 Stat. 1330 (1987).

Institute of Medicine's Committee on Nursing Home Regulation which found that, at the time, quality of care in many of the nation's nursing homes was lacking.[136] The Committee on Nursing Home Regulation therefore recommended "[a] major reorientation of the regulatory system is needed to make it focus on the care being provided to residents and the effects of the care on their well-being."[137]

The Act required SNFs and NFs to provide, among other things, "services to attain or maintain the highest practicable physical, mental, and psychosocial well-being of each resident, in accordance with a written plan of care[,]"[138]and established minimum personnel requirements for resident nursing care.[139] The Act also included a resident "bill of rights" requiring NFs and SNFs to promote and protect the rights of residents to, among other things, be free from restraints, including chemical restraints, imposed for discipline or convenience and the rights of residents to be active participants in the planning of their medical care.[140] In furtherance of the Act's intent and policy objectives, the HCFA[141] issued implementing regulations in 1989 and 1991, establishing the Conditions of Participation (CoPs) for SNFs and NFs participating in the Medicare and Medicaid programs.[142] However, enforcement of some implementing regulations did not become effective until July 1995, attributable, in part, to the large volume of comments HCFA received during the rulemaking process.[143]

On July 16, 2015, CMS issued a proposed rule to update comprehensively the CoPs for NFs and SNFs participating in the Medicare and Medicaid programs. CMS issued its final rule on October 4, 2016.[144]

---

[136] INST. OF MED., COMM. ON NURSING HOME REGULATION, IMPROVING THE QUALITY OF CARE IN NURSING HOMES 22 (1986). *See also* U.S. GEN. ACCOUNTING OFFICE, GAO/HEHS-99-46, Nursing Homes: Additional Steps Needed to Strengthen Enforcement of Federal Quality Standards 5 (1999) *available at* https://www.gao.gov/assets/230/227015.pdf.

[137] INST. OF MED., *supra* note 90 at 22.

[138] 42 U.S.C. § 1395i-3(b)(2) and 42 U.S.C. § 1396r(b)(2) (Under the Act, NFs must also provide residents activities in accordance with the written plan of care).

[139] 42 U.S.C. §§ 1395i-3(b)(4)-(5) and 42 U.S.C. §§ 1396r(b) (4)-(5).

[140] 42 U.S.C. § 1395i-3(c) and 42 U.S.C. § 1396r(c).

[141] The HCFA was renamed the Centers for Medicare & Medicaid Services (CMS) in June 2001. *See* CNN, *supra* note 60.

[142] 54 Fed. Reg. 5,316 (Feb. 2, 1989) and 56 Fed. Reg. 48,826 (Sept. 26, 1991).

[143] U.S. Gen. Accounting Office, *supra* note 90.

[144] 81 Fed. Reg. 68,688 (Oct. 4, 2016).

The final rule divided the updated CoPs into three phases—with Phase 1 requirements to be implemented by November 28, 2016 and Phase 2 and Phase 3 requirements to be implemented by November 28, 2017 and November 28, 2019, respectively.[145] CMS estimated that the total projected cost of the final rule would be $831 million in the first year of implementation, and $736 million per year in subsequent years.[146]

In a June 30, 2017 memorandum, CMS announced that it was imposing a 12-month moratorium on the use of civil money penalties, denial of payment, and/or termination from the Medicare and Medicaid programs, for facilities determined to be out-of-compliance with certain Phase 2 regulations, though noting that the regulations would still take effect on November 28, 2017.[147] CMS maintained that it would use the year-long period to "educate facilities about certain new Phase 2 quality standards by requiring a directed plan of correction or additional in-service training."[148] On November 24, 2017, CMS announced it was extending the moratorium on the enforcement of certain Phase 2 requirements for a period of 18-months, in lieu of the previously announced 12-months, "[t]o address concerns regarding the scope and timing of the revised requirements[.]"[149]

Issues

The following issues may be examined at the hearing:

---

[145] *Id.*

[146] *Id.*

[147] Memorandum from Dir., Survey and Certification Group, Centers for Medicare and Medicaid Services to State Survey Agency Directors (June 30, 2017) *available at* https://www.cms.gov/Medicare/Provider-Enrollment-and-Certification/SurveyCertificationGenInfo/Downloads/Survey-and-Cert-Letter-17-36.pdf.

[148] *Id.*

[149] Memorandum from Dir., Survey and Certification Group, Centers for Medicare and Medicaid Services to State Survey Agency Directors (Nov. 24, 2017) *available at* https://www.cms.gov/Medicare/Provider-Enrollment-and-Certification/SurveyCertificationGenInfo/Downloads/Survey-and-Cert-Letter-18-04.pdf. In its memo, CMS noted that it was not extending the moratorium on regulations that address reporting requirements for the reasonable suspicion of a crime due to the concerns about significant resident abuse going unreported.

- Federal efforts to verify that SNFs and NFs participating in the Medicare and Medicaid programs are meeting the mandatory CoPs, which are intended to ensure that beneficiaries receive the appropriate levels of care and are free from abuse or neglect;
- The role of State Survey Agencies in overseeing SNFs and NFs, and CMS' oversight thereof;
- The consistency and proportionality of enforcement remedies imposed on SNFs and NFs that have been determined to be out of compliance with one or more CoPs;
- Evaluation of SNFs and NFs that have a commonality of ownership;
- CMS' Administration of the Special Focus Facility program;
- Implementation of the emergency preparedness rule and the adequacy of emergency preparedness in SNFs and NFs across the country; and
- HHS OIG's and GAO's work evaluating abuse, neglect, and substandard care occurring at SNFs and NFs.

In: Nursing Homes and Elder Abuse
Editor: Joshua Newland
ISBN: 978-1-53617-974-3
© 2020 Nova Science Publishers, Inc.

Chapter 2

NURSING HOMES: IMPROVED OVERSIGHT NEEDED TO BETTER PROTECT RESIDENTS FROM ABUSE*

United States Government Accountability Office

ABBREVIATIONS

CMS	Centers for Medicare & Medicaid Services
HHS	Department of Health and Human Services
OIG	Office of Inspector General
MFCU	Medicaid Fraud Control Unit

WHY GAO DID THIS STUDY

Nursing homes provide care to about 1.4 million nursing home residents—a vulnerable population of elderly and disabled individuals.

* This is an edited, reformatted and augmented version of United States Government Accountability Office; Report to Congressional Requesters, Publication No. GAO-19-433, dated June 2019.

CMS, an agency within the Department of Health and Human Services (HHS), defines standards nursing homes must meet to participate in the Medicare and Medicaid programs.

GAO was asked to review abuse of residents in nursing homes. Among other objectives, this report: (1) determines the trends and types of abuse in recent years, and (2) evaluates CMS oversight intended to ensure residents are free from abuse.

GAO reviewed CMS's policies, analyzed CMS data on abuse deficiencies from 2013 through 2017, the most recent data at the time of our review, and interviewed officials from CMS and state survey agencies in five states, as well as other key stakeholders in those states such as ombudsmen and law enforcement officials. The states were selected for variation in factors such as number of nursing homes and role of other state agencies in abuse investigations.

What GAO Recommends

GAO is making six recommendations, including that CMS: require state survey agencies to submit data on abuse and perpetrator type; require state survey agencies to immediately refer to law enforcement any suspicion of a crime; and develop guidance on what abuse information nursing homes should self-report. HHS concurred with all of GAO's recommendations and

What GAO Found

The Centers for Medicare & Medicaid Services (CMS) is responsible for ensuring nursing homes meet federal quality standards, including that residents are free from abuse. CMS enters into agreements with state survey agencies to conduct surveys of the state's homes and to investigate complaints and incidents. GAO analysis of CMS data found that, while relatively rare, abuse deficiencies cited in nursing homes more than doubled, increasing from 430 in 2013 to 875 in 2017, with the largest increase in severe cases. GAO also reviewed a representative sample of abuse deficiency narratives from 2016 through 2017. Physical and mental/verbal abuse occurred most often in nursing homes, followed by sexual abuse, and staff were more often the perpetrators of the abuse deficiencies cited. CMS cannot readily access information on abuse or perpetrator type in its data and, therefore, lacks key information critical to taking appropriate actions.

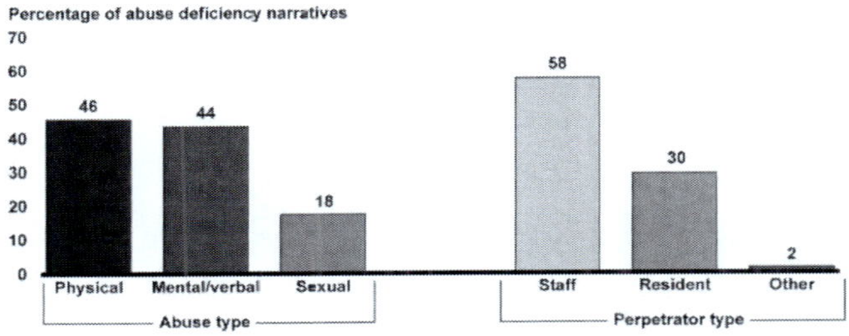

Source: GAO analysis of Centers for Medicare & Medicaid Services' (CMS) data and supporting narratives. | GAO-19-433

Note: Percentages do not add to 100 because some narratives had multiple types of abuse, were missing or incomplete, or were not consistent with CMS's definition of abuse.

GAO Analysis of a Representative Sample of CMS Nursing Home Abuse Deficiency Narratives, 2016-2017.

GAO also found gaps in CMS oversight, including:

- Gaps in CMS processes that can result in delayed and missed referrals. Federal law requires nursing home staff to immediately report to law enforcement and the state survey agency reasonable suspicions of a crime that results in serious bodily injury to a resident. However, there is no equivalent requirement that the state survey agency make a timely referral for complaints it receives directly or through surveys it conducts. CMS also does not conduct oversight to ensure that state survey agencies are correctly referring abuse cases to law enforcement.

- Insufficient information collected on facility-reported incidents. CMS has not issued guidance on what nursing homes should include when they self-report abuse incidents to the state survey agencies. Officials from all of the state survey agencies in GAO's review said the facility-reported incidents can lack information needed to prioritize investigations and may result in state survey agencies not responding as quickly as needed.

June 13, 2019

The Honorable Chuck Grassley
Chairman

The Honorable Ron Wyden
Ranking Member
Committee on Finance
United States Senate

The Honorable Rob Portman
Chairman

The Honorable Thomas Carper
Ranking Member
Permanent Subcommittee on Investigations
Committee on Homeland Security and Governmental Affairs
United States Senate

Nationwide, more than 15,500 nursing homes participating in the Medicare and Medicaid programs provide care to about 1.4 million elderly or disabled nursing home residents. These residents often have physical and cognitive limitations that can make them particularly vulnerable to abuse. Abuse of nursing home residents can occur in many forms—including physical, mental, verbal, and sexual—and can be committed by staff, residents, or others in the nursing home. Little is known about the full scope of nursing home abuse, as incidents of abuse may be underreported.[1] Any incident of abuse is a serious occurrence and could result in potentially devastating consequences for residents, including lasting mental anguish, serious injury, or death.

Federal law mandates that nursing homes receiving Medicare and Medicaid payments must ensure that residents are free from abuse. To help ensure this, the Centers for Medicare & Medicaid Services (CMS), an agency within the Department of Health and Human Services (HHS), defines the quality standards that nursing homes must meet in order to participate in the Medicare and Medicaid programs.[2] To monitor compliance with these standards, CMS enters into agreements with agencies in each state government—known as state survey agencies— and oversees the work the state survey agencies do.[3] This work includes conducting required evaluations—referred to as standard surveys—approximately once each year of all nursing homes in a state that participate in the Medicare or Medicaid programs, as well as investigating both complaints from the public and facility-reported incidents regarding resident care or safety.[4] When a state survey agency finds a nursing home

---

[1] C. Hawes, *Elder Abuse in Residential Long-Term Care Settings: What is Known and What Information is Needed?* National Research Council of the National Academies, Panel to Review Risk and Prevalence of Elder Abuse and Neglect. (Washington, D.C.: 2003).

[2] CMS defines abuse in its guidance, the State Operations Manual (dated November 22, 2017), as: "The willful infliction of injury, unreasonable confinement, intimidation, or punishment with resulting physical harm, pain or mental anguish. Abuse also includes the deprivation by an individual, including a caretaker, of goods or services that are necessary to attain or maintain physical, mental, and psychosocial well-being." This report addresses physical abuse, mental and verbal abuse—which we refer to as "mental/verbal abuse"— and sexual abuse but does not address other forms of abuse, such as financial abuse or neglect.
Medicare, the federal health insurance program for people age 65 and older, individuals under age 65 with certain disabilities, and individuals diagnosed with end-stage renal disease, covers some short-term skilled nursing and rehabilitative care for beneficiaries following an acute care hospital stay. Medicaid, a joint federal-state health program for low-income and medically needy individuals, is the nation's primary payer of long-term services and supports for children and adults with disabilities and aged individuals.

[3] Survey agencies are frequently housed in the human services department of state governments and may have different names in different states.

[4] By law, every nursing home receiving Medicare or Medicaid payment must undergo a standard survey during which teams of state surveyors conduct a comprehensive on-site evaluation of compliance with federal quality standards. These surveys must occur at least once every fifteen months, with a statewide average interval for surveys not to exceed 12 months. 42 U.S.C. §§ 1395i-3(g)(1)(A), (g)(2)(A)(iii), 1396r(g)(1)(A), (g)(2)(A)(iii).

out of compliance with a federal standard, the home receives a deficiency citation, also known as a deficiency.

In addition to state survey agencies, other state-based agencies are charged with protecting nursing home residents from abuse. These agencies' roles, missions, and standards of evidence for determining whether or not abuse occurred can vary by state. For example, Adult Protective Services may also help ensure nursing home residents receive quality care in a safe environment by investigating allegations of abuse.[5] Law enforcement can also play a role in protecting nursing home residents from abuse and, in addition, Medicaid Fraud Control Units (MFCU) in each state are tasked with investigating and prosecuting a variety of health care-related crimes.

We have previously reported on problems in nursing home quality, including problems protecting residents from abuse and weaknesses in CMS's oversight. For example, in multiple reports dating back to 1998, we have identified weaknesses in federal and state activities designed to correct quality problems in nursing homes. Specifically, in a 2002 report, we found that CMS needed to do more to protect nursing home residents from abuse and made five recommendations to help CMS facilitate the reporting, investigation, and prevention of abuse in nursing homes.[6] More recently, in April 2019 we reported that CMS had failed to address gaps in federal oversight of nursing home abuse investigations in Oregon that persisted for at least 15 years until the Oregon state survey agency changed

State survey agencies are also required to investigate allegations of neglect and abuse in nursing homes in response to complaints and facility-reported incidents filed with state survey agencies. 42 U.S.C. §§ 1395i-3(g)(1)(C), 1396r(g)(1)(C). During an investigation, state surveyors evaluate the nursing home's compliance with a specific federal quality standard.

[5] Long-term care ombudsmen and Adult Protective Services may investigate and resolve complaints involving residents of nursing homes. In some states, Adult Protective Services may not have jurisdiction in nursing homes. While Adult Protective Services operates at the state level, some states receive federal funding for part or all of their programs.

[6] One of our recommendations was implemented—that CMS clarify the definition of abuse and otherwise ensure that states apply that definition consistently and appropriately. While CMS generally agreed with our recommendations, the other four recommendations were closed as not implemented. See GAO, *Nursing Homes: More Can Be Done to Protect Residents from Abuse*, GAO-02-312, (Washington, D.C.: March 1, 2002).

its practices in October 2018.[7] Further, a 2017 HHS Office of the Inspector General (OIG) report found that CMS does not have adequate procedures in place to ensure incidents of potential abuse in nursing homes are identified and reported.[8] In addition, news reports have described concerning examples of incidents where nursing home residents were abused.[9]

You asked us to review abuse of nursing home residents including, among other issues, what CMS data reveal about the prevalence of abuse and the extent to which CMS oversees nursing homes. In this report, we:

1. determine the trends and types of abuse occurring in nursing homes in recent years,
2. describe the risk factors for abuse and challenges facing stakeholder agencies involved in investigating abuse in nursing homes, and
3. evaluate CMS oversight intended to ensure that nursing home residents are free from abuse.

To determine the trends and types of abuse occurring in nursing homes in recent years, we reviewed CMS guidance and analyzed CMS data from 2013 through 2017, which represented the most recent data for a 5-year period at the time of our review. First, we reviewed the CMS State Operations Manual in effect during our period of review to determine the federal standards and associated deficiency codes related to resident abuse.[10] We focused our analysis on the deficiency code to be used by state

---

[7] GAO, *Management Report: CMS Needs to Address Gaps in Federal Oversight of Nursing Home Abuse Investigations That Persisted in Oregon for at Least 15 Years,* GAO-19-313R (Washington, D.C.: Apr. 15, 2019).

[8] See Daniel R. Levinson, OIG, HHS, memorandum to Seema Verma, Administrator, CMS, *Early Alert: The Centers for Medicare & Medicaid Services Has Inadequate Procedures To Ensure That Incidents of Potential Abuse or Neglect at Skilled Nursing Facilities Are Identified and Reported in Accordance With Applicable Requirements*, A-01-17-00504 (Washington, D.C.: August 24, 2017).

[9] For example, see Blake Ellis and Melanie Hicken, "Sick, Dying, and Raped in America's Nursing Homes," CNN, February 22, 2017. Also see Chris Serres, "Left to Suffer: A Five-Part Series," Minneapolis Star Tribune, November 12, 2017.

[10] Specifically, we reviewed Appendix PP of the State Operations Manual because it is the section that provides guidance to state surveyors about determining compliance with federal

surveyors when a nursing home fails to keep a resident free from abuse, which encompasses mental/verbal, sexual, or physical abuse.[11]

We analyzed data provided by CMS to identify the number and severity of abuse deficiencies cited by surveyors in all 50 states and Washington D.C. between 2013 and 2017. We then tracked (1) whether these abuse deficiencies originated from a standard survey, complaint investigation, or facility-reported incident investigation and (2) the enforcement actions associated with these abuse deficiencies. Furthermore, we determined the number of nursing homes that had one or more abuse deficiencies from 2013 through 2017, as well as the homes with repeated abuse deficiencies in multiple years and the characteristics of those homes.[12]

Finally, because abuse and perpetrator type are not readily identifiable in CMS's data, we identified this information by reviewing a randomly selected representative sample of 400 abuse deficiency narratives written by state surveyors from 2016 through 2017 that describe the substantiated abuse. Specifically, two separate reviewers independently analyzed the text of each narrative and determined if the abuse was physical, mental/verbal, or sexual and whether the perpetrators were staff, residents, or others based on narrative descriptions written by state surveyors.[13] Any disagreements between the two reviewers were resolved by a third independent reviewer. We assessed the reliability of each of the datasets by checking for missing

---

quality standards and their associated deficiency codes. There were multiple updates to Appendix PP of the State Operations Manual during the period of our review (January 1, 2013, through November 27, 2017). Specifically, there were eight updates to the appendix during the 5-year period, but none of these changed the abuse deficiency citation codes used by state surveyors. Therefore, we used the March 8, 2017, version of the Appendix PP—the most recent version during our period of review—when determining which deficiency codes to analyze for this report. CMS, *State Operations Manual, Appendix PP—Guidance to Surveyors for Long Term Care Facilities.* (March 8, 2017).

CMS restructured its deficiency code system beginning on November 28, 2017, and, due to these coding changes, we did not analyze CMS data cited by surveyors after the implementation of that change.

[11] For the purposes of this report, we refer to mental and verbal abuse as "mental/verbal abuse." Over the period of time examined in our review, CMS's abuse deficiency code also included involuntary seclusion.

[12] For the purposes of this report, we include Washington, D.C. when we refer to data for states.

[13] We analyzed the abuse deficiency narratives according to CMS's definitions in its State Operations Manual. CMS, *State Operations Manual, Appendix PP—Guidance to Surveyors for Long Term Care Facilities*. (November 22, 2017).

values and obvious errors and discussing them with CMS officials who were knowledgeable about the data. In the course of this assessment, we found some data limitations. Specifically, CMS officials told us that some state survey agencies may not have entered all facility-reported incidents into the CMS database while other state survey agencies did.[14] In a recent 2019 report, we also found that the Oregon state survey agency was not entering all abuse-related complaints or facility-reported incidents into the CMS database—a problem that could exist in other states.[15] In addition, CMS officials told us that it is possible there are additional incidents that may not have been represented in the abuse deficiency data during the period of our review. Specifically, CMS officials noted that some incidents resulting from resident altercations—particularly those that do not show a willful intent to harm—may not be cited as an abuse deficiency by some state survey agencies. We therefore consider the number of abuse deficiencies that resulted from complaints or facility-reported incidents to be a conservative estimate. After reviewing the possible limitations of these data, we determined the data were sufficiently reliable for the purposes of this reporting objective. (See app. I for additional details on the scope and methodology of our data analyses.)

To describe the risk factors for abuse and challenges facing stakeholder agencies involved in investigating abuse in nursing homes, we interviewed officials from a non-generalizable sample of five state survey agencies—Delaware, Georgia, Ohio, Oregon, and Virginia. We selected these states for variation in geography, whether the states' Adult Protective Services has oversight over nursing home residents, the number of nursing homes in each state, CMS regional oversight, and congressional interest. In addition to speaking to officials from state survey agencies, we interviewed other stakeholders in these states, including officials from each state's long-term care ombudsmen, law enforcement, MFCUs, and, when appropriate, Adult

---

[14] CMS guidance requires state survey agencies to enter facility-reported incidents into the CMS database that require a federal, on-site survey.

[15] See GAO-19-313R. Further, our 2011 report noted CMS's concerns regarding the underreporting of complaints from state survey agencies. See GAO, *Nursing Homes: More Reliable Data and Consistent Guidance Would Improve CMS Oversight of State Complaint Investigations*, GAO-11-280, (Washington, D.C.: Apr. 7, 2011).

Protective Services.[16] We also visited nursing homes and spoke to administrators and clinical staff in each state. We selected these nursing homes to obtain variation in factors such as bed count and profit or not-for-profit status. We asked stakeholders to describe the risk factors for abuse and the challenges involved in investigating abuse in nursing homes. In addition, we interviewed officials from national organizations with knowledge of nursing home abuse issues including the American Health Care Association, National Consumer Voice, and the National Adult Protective Services Association to learn more about the risk factors for abuse and the challenges facing stakeholders involved in investigating abuse.

To evaluate CMS oversight intended to ensure that nursing home residents are free from abuse, we reviewed relevant federal laws and CMS guidance, such as the State Operations Manual, that establishes CMS and state survey agency oversight responsibilities for nursing homes. We also interviewed officials at the CMS central office, the CMS regional offices that oversee the five state survey agencies in our review, and the five state survey agencies themselves. We assessed CMS's oversight activities in the context of the federal standards for internal control related to information and communications and monitoring.[17]

We conducted this performance audit from October 2017 to June 2019 in accordance with generally accepted government auditing standards. Those standards require that we plan and perform the audit to obtain sufficient, appropriate evidence to provide a reasonable basis for our findings and conclusions based on our audit objectives. We believe that the evidence obtained provides a reasonable basis for our findings and conclusions based on our audit objectives.

---

[16] We only interviewed officials from Adult Protective Services in Oregon and Virginia because, in those states, Adult Protective Services had nursing home oversight whereas in the other states in our review, it did not.

[17] GAO, *Standards for Internal Control in the Federal Government*. GAO-14-704G (Washington, D.C.: Sept. 10, 2014). Internal control is a process effected by an entity's oversight body, management, and other personnel that provides reasonable assurance that the objectives of an entity will be achieved.

BACKGROUND

Nursing homes are required to keep residents safe from harm, but when abuse is alleged, a combination of federal, state, and local agencies—as well as the nursing homes themselves—play a role in investigating.

Federal Oversight of Nursing Homes

Federal laws establish minimum requirements nursing homes must meet to participate in the Medicare and Medicaid programs, including standards for the quality of care.[18] These standards cover a variety of categories, such as resident rights, quality of care, and quality of life. In 2016, CMS finalized a comprehensive update to its nursing home standards to reflect new requirements and align requirements with current clinical practices, among other things. The changes were implemented in three phases, starting November 28, 2016.[19]

The federal government and the states share oversight responsibility for the nation's nursing homes, with specific activities occurring at the national, regional, and state levels.

- CMS central office. At the national level, the CMS central office oversees the federal standards nursing homes must meet to participate in the Medicare and Medicaid programs. Primarily through its State Operations Manual, the office establishes the responsibilities of CMS's regional offices and state survey

[18] Titles XVIII and XIX of the Social Security Act, as amended, establish minimum requirements nursing homes must meet to participate in the Medicare and Medicaid programs, respectively.
The Social Security Act and their implementing regulations use the terms "skilled nursing facility" (Medicare) and "nursing facility" (Medicaid). For the purposes of this report, we use the term nursing home to refer to both skilled nursing facilities and nursing facilities.

[19] Medicare and Medicaid Programs; Reform of Requirements for Long-Term Care Facilities, 81 Fed. Reg. 686888 (Oct. 4, 2016).Phase 1 (effective November 28, 2016) implemented most minor modifications to the existing nursing home regulations; phase 2 (effective November 28, 2017) implemented new regulations and re-structured CMS's deficiency code system; and phase 3 (effective November 28, 2019) will implement the remaining requirements.

agencies in ensuring that federal quality standards for nursing homes are met.

- CMS regional offices. CMS's 10 regional offices oversee state activities and report back to the CMS central office the results of their efforts. Specifically, regional offices use the State Performance Standards System to evaluate state surveyors' performance on factors such as the frequency and quality of state surveys.
- State survey agencies. Under agreement with CMS, a state survey agency in each state assesses whether nursing homes meet CMS's standards, allowing them to participate in the Medicare and Medicaid programs. State survey agencies assess nursing homes using (1) recurring standard surveys and (2) as-needed investigations.
  - Standard surveys. State survey agencies are required by federal law to perform unannounced, on-site standard surveys of every nursing home receiving Medicare or Medicaid payment at least every 15 months, with a statewide average frequency of every 12 months. These surveys are a comprehensive assessment designed to determine whether nursing homes are complying with Medicare and Medicaid quality standards.[20]
  - Investigations. In addition to standard surveys, state survey agencies are required by federal law to investigate (1) complaints submitted by residents, family members, friends, physicians, and nursing home staff; and (2) "facility-reported incidents," including incidents involving abuse of residents, that are self-reported by the nursing homes. State survey agencies review the information provided through these

---

[20] On November 28, 2017, as a part of implementation phase 2, CMS rolled out a new survey system—which implemented our 2015 recommendation that CMS establish timeframes for the development and implementation of a standardized survey system across all states. The new survey system was implemented simultaneously nationwide, so that all states are now using the same survey system when, prior to the change, states were split between two different survey systems, complicating assessments of nursing home quality. See GAO, *Nursing Home Quality: CMS Should Continue to Improve Data and Oversight*, GAO-16-33 (Washington, D.C.: Oct. 30, 2015).

complaints and incidents and determine if an on-site investigation is required. During this unannounced investigation, the state surveyors assess available evidence to determine whether the allegation can be substantiated. These investigations offer the state survey agency the opportunity to identify and correct care problems in a more timely manner than through the standard surveys.

If a surveyor determines that a nursing home violated a federal standard during a survey or investigation, then a deficiency code specific to that standard is cited. For instance, one deficiency code for abuse of residents encompasses mental/verbal, sexual, or physical abuse; while a few additional deficiency codes encompass abuse-related issues, such as a failure by the nursing home to train staff on issues related to abuse. Cited deficiencies are then classified into categories according to scope (the number of residents potentially affected) and severity (the potential for or occurrence of harm to residents). (See Table 1.) State survey agencies are required to enter data about deficiencies into CMS's survey database. For most deficiencies, the nursing home is required to prepare a plan of correction, and, depending on the scope and severity of the deficiency, surveyors may re-visit the facility to ensure that the nursing home has implemented its plan and corrected the deficiency. In any instances where surveyors substantiate the occurrence of resident abuse, the state survey agency is required to refer the case to three entities: 1) local law enforcement; 2) the MFCU, if appropriate; and 3) the state's nurse aide registry or other applicable professional licensure authority.[21]

When nursing homes are cited with deficiencies, federal enforcement actions—or penalties—can be imposed to encourage homes to make corrections. In general, enforcement actions: (1) may be initially recommended by the state survey agency, (2) are transferred to the CMS regional office for review, (3) are imposed by the same CMS regional office, and (4) are implemented—that is, put into effect. Depending on the

[21] In nursing homes, the primary caregivers are nurse aides.

scope and severity of the deficiency cited, the CMS regional office may impose certain enforcement actions so that they are implemented immediately. However, for other enforcement actions, the regional office may provide the nursing home with an opportunity to correct the deficiencies, which, if corrected before the scheduled effective date, can result in the penalty not being implemented. Penalties include directed in-service training, fines known as civil money penalties, denial of payment, and termination from the Medicare and Medicaid programs, among others. (See Figure 1.)

Reporting and Investigation of Abuse by Nursing Homes

When a nursing home becomes aware of an incident of alleged resident abuse, the home must: immediately report the allegation to the state survey agency and then conduct an investigation of the alleged incident. Specifically, the process is as follows:

Table 1. Centers for Medicare & Medicaid Services' (CMS) Alphabetical Scope and Severity Categories for Nursing Home Deficiencies

Severity	Isolated	Pattern	Widespread
No actual harm with a potential for minimal harm[a]	A	B	C
No actual harm with a potential for more than minimal harm	D	E	F
Actual harm	G	H	I
Immediate jeopardy[b]	J	K	L

Source: CMS. | GAO-19-433.

[a] Nursing home is considered to be in "substantial compliance."

[b] Caused, or is likely to cause, serious injury, harm, impairment, or death.

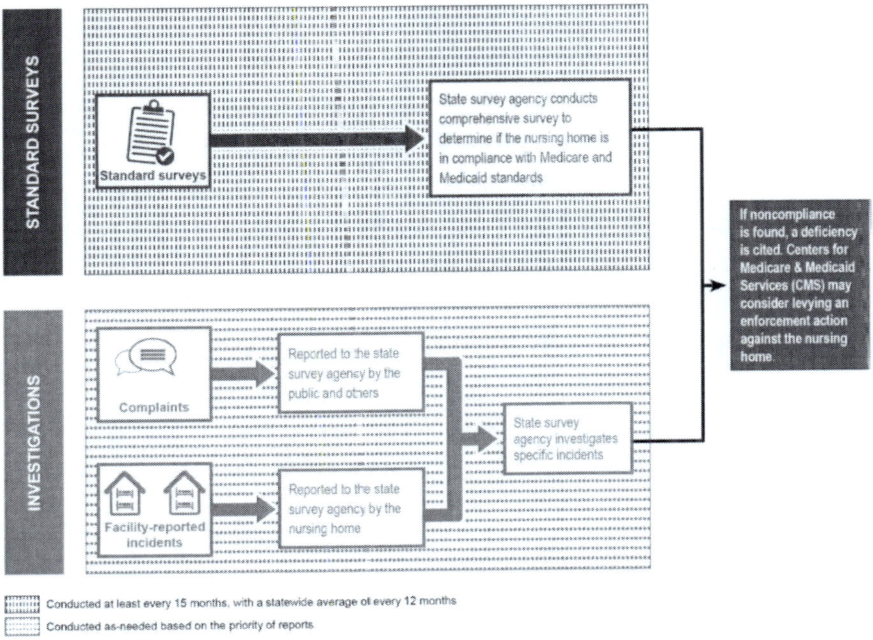

Source: GAO summary of CMS policies. | GAO-19-433

Figure 1. Primary Methods Used by State Survey Agencies to Assess Whether Nursing Homes Are Meeting Federal Standards.

- The nursing home must immediately report alleged abuse to the state survey agency. After notifying the state survey agency, the nursing home is also required to conduct its own investigation and submit its findings in a written report to the state survey agency within 5 working days of the incident.
- Depending on the severity of the circumstances, the state survey agency may visit the nursing home to investigate the incident or wait until the nursing home submits its report.
- Depending on the content of the report, the state survey agency may request the home conduct additional work or the state survey agency may investigate further on its own.
- If the state survey agency opts not to investigate further, it may still review the manner in which the home conducted its

investigation during the state survey agency's next scheduled standard survey.

- If a state survey agency determines that a nurse aide is responsible for abuse, the agency must add this finding to the state's nurse aide registry—a registry that each state is required to maintain that lists all individuals who have satisfactorily completed approved nurse aide training and a competency evaluation program in that state.[22] Nursing homes are prohibited from employing a nurse aide with a finding of abuse on the nurse aide registry.
- Further, if there is a reasonable suspicion that a crime has occurred that results in serious bodily injury, federal law requires certain covered individuals at the nursing home to immediately report to law enforcement in addition to the state survey agency.[23]

Before employing a nurse aide, nursing homes are required to check each relevant state's registry to verify that the nurse aide has passed a competency evaluation. All nursing homes must also verify with the relevant state board of licensing the professional credentials of the licensed personnel, such as registered nurses, whom they hire.[24]

Other State and Local Agencies that May Investigate Abuse in Nursing Homes

In addition to state survey agencies, there are other state and local agencies that may be involved in investigating abuse in nursing homes.

---

[22] 42 C.F.R. § 483.156 (2018).

[23] 42 U.S.C. § 1320b-25(b). This is known as the 1150(b) requirement after its location in the Social Security Act. These covered individuals include nursing home owners, operators, and employees, among others.

[24] In contrast, state survey agencies are not responsible for disciplining other nursing home professionals, such as registered nurses, who are suspected of abuse. However, such personnel are referred by the state survey agency to their respective state licensing boards for review and possible disciplinary action.

These other state and local agencies that investigate abuse in nursing homes are generally focused on the different aspects of the specific alleged abuse incident, in contrast to the state survey agency, which focuses on the safety of individual residents, as well as on the facility's policies and procedures for preventing and effectively addressing abuse. These other state and local agencies include:

- Adult Protective Services. In some states, Adult Protective Services' investigators are trained to provide protection and intervention for older adults in nursing homes and can play a valuable role in helping to protect residents from abuse.[25]
- Ombudsmen. Long-term care ombudsmen, who serve as advocates for nursing home residents, may also investigate abuse complaints made by or on behalf of residents.
- Local law enforcement. Law enforcement may also play a role in investigating alleged nursing home resident abuse. Specifically, local police departments may learn of suspected instances of resident abuse and conduct criminal investigations.
- MFCU. The state MFCUs typically learn of abuse allegations through referrals from state survey agencies, which CMS requires if abuse is substantiated. If, after investigating an allegation, the MFCU decides that there is sufficient evidence to press criminal charges, it may prosecute the case itself or refer the matter to the state's attorney general or a local prosecutor.

---

[25] Adult Protective Services is generally responsible for identifying, investigating, resolving, and preventing abuse of older adults, although in some states, Adult Protective Services may not have jurisdiction in nursing homes. For more information, see GAO, *Elder Justice. Stronger Federal Leadership Could Enhance National Response to Elder Abuse*, GAO-11-208 (Washington, D.C.: Mar. 2, 2011).
In addition, the Administration for Community Living within HHS collects Adult Protective Services data voluntarily submitted by states as part of its National Adult Maltreatment Reporting System. The first year of data submission was federal fiscal year 2016.

MORE ABUSE DEFICIENCIES WERE CITED IN NURSING HOMES FROM 2013 THROUGH 2017; PHYSICAL AND MENTAL/VERBAL ABUSE AND STAFF PERPETRATORS WERE MOST COMMON

Abuse Deficiencies Cited and the Number of Nursing Homes Involved More than Doubled from 2013 through 2017, with the Largest Increase in Severe Cases

Our analysis of CMS data found that from 2013 through 2017, abuse deficiencies cited in nursing homes became more frequent, with the largest increase in severe cases.[26] While abuse deficiencies are relatively rare—they comprise less than 1 percent of the total deficiencies in each of the years we examined—they became more common over the 5-year period. Specifically, the number of abuse deficiencies cited more than doubled—from 430 in 2013 to 875 in 2017 (a 103.5 percent increase).[27] This trend for the abuse deficiencies is in contrast to the trend for all deficiencies, which decreased about 1 percent between 2013 and 2017.[28] At the state level, 32 states had more abuse deficiencies cited in 2017 than 2013, six states had a consistent number, and the remaining 13 had fewer. (See app. III for additional data on abuse deficiencies by state.) Furthermore, abuse deficiencies cited in 2017 were more likely to be categorized at the highest levels of severity—deficiencies causing actual harm to residents or putting

---

[26] We analyzed the deficiency code cited when state surveyors determine that a nursing home failed to keep a resident free from abuse, which encompasses mental/verbal, sexual, or physical abuse. An abuse deficiency may represent a single incident of abuse with one perpetrator and one victim; however, an abuse deficiency could also encompass multiple incidents of abuse with more than one perpetrator and victim.

[27] The total average number of nursing home residents in surveyed nursing homes decreased slightly, by less than 1 percent—from about 1,258,089 in 2013 to 1,249,970 in 2017.

[28] All deficiency types increased at a much slower rate than abuse deficiencies through 2016 and then decreased slightly through the period examined in 2017.
We also found an increasing trend in abuse-related deficiencies—that is, a nursing home's failure to have proper policies in place to protect residents from abuse, such as established procedures to report and investigate alleged mistreatment, neglect, or abuse and to train staff on issues related to abuse—cited in nursing homes from 2013 through 2017. Specifically, abuse-related deficiencies increased by 9.9 percent over the 5-year period, from 4,899 deficiencies in 2013 to 5,383 deficiencies in 2017. See appendix II for more information.

residents in immediate jeopardy—than they were in 2013.[29] Specifically, 42.6 percent of the 875 abuse deficiencies were categorized as causing actual harm or posing immediate jeopardy to residents in 2017, compared to 31.9 percent of the 430 abuse deficiencies in 2013. (See Figure 2.)

In examining the types of survey or investigations conducted to identify abuse deficiencies, we found that, from 2013 to 2017, the majority (about two-thirds in each year) were identified through either a complaint investigation or facility-reported incident investigation.[30] In contrast, for all types of deficiencies, we found the inverse—the vast majority were identified through a standard survey. This demonstrates the unique and significant role that complaint and facility-reported incident investigations have in identifying abuse deficiencies, because they allow for the identification and correction of abuse in a more timely manner than a standard survey. In fact, for the deficiencies for which we were able to identify the source, the percentage of abuse deficiencies identified through facility-reported incident investigations increased from 42.3 percent of the 430 abuse deficiencies in 2013 to 47.4 percent of the 875 abuse deficiencies in 2017.[31] Conversely, for all types of deficiencies, a very small percentage resulted from facility-reported incident investigations—about 5 percent or less each year. (See Figure 3.)

---

[29] Abuse deficiencies were categorized by scope—whether the incident was an isolated occurrence, a part of a pattern of behavior, or a widespread behavior—consistently each year, with about 82 percent of abuse deficiencies cited categorized as isolated, about 15 percent categorized as a pattern, and about 3 percent categorized as widespread.

[30] We found that some deficiencies were identified through a combination of complaint investigations, facility-reported incident investigations, standard surveys, or all three. For instance, a family member could submit a complaint about an alleged abuse incident, and the facility could self-report that same incident, leading to a single investigation and abuse deficiency. We counted those deficiencies as originating from each relevant category.
We also became aware that while CMS guidance requires all complaints to be entered into its database, it does not require state survey agencies to enter all facility-reported incidents—only those that require a federal, on-site survey. As a result, our estimate may be conservative.

[31] For 375 out of 2,892 abuse deficiencies and 55,190 out of 538,559 total deficiencies cited over the 5-year time period, we were unable to determine from CMS's data whether the deficiency was identified during a standard survey, complaint investigation, facility-reported incident investigation, or a combination. We excluded these deficiencies from our percentages.

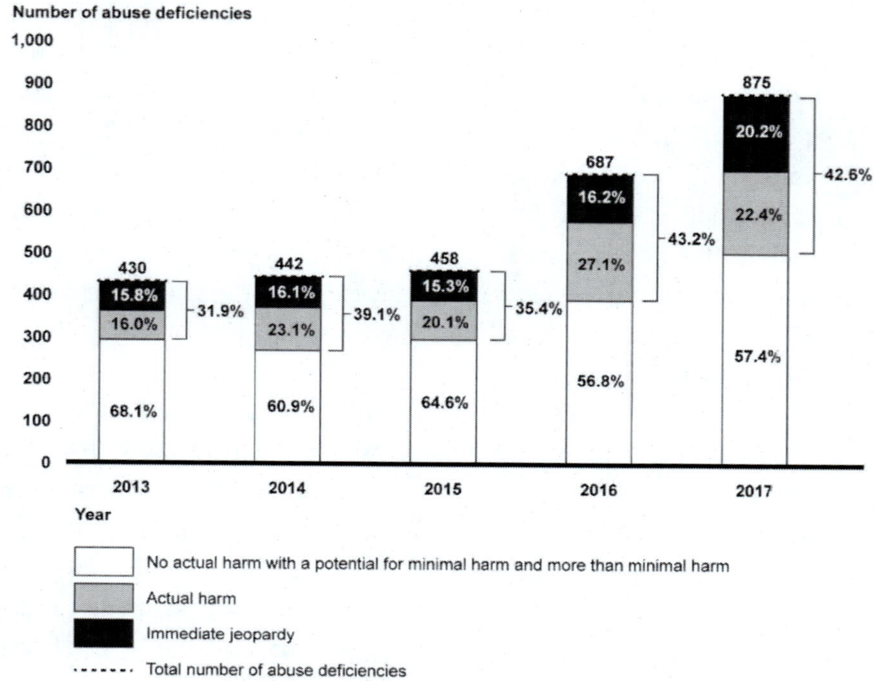

Source: GAO analysis of Centers for Medicare & Medicaid Services' (CMS) data. | GAO-19-433

Notes: CMS categorizes deficiencies into one of four severity categories based on whether the deficiency constitutes: (1) no actual harm with a potential for minimal harm; (2) no actual harm with a potential for more than minimal harm, but not immediate jeopardy; (3) actual harm that is not immediate jeopardy; or (4) immediate jeopardy to resident health or safety. We combined the first two categories in this figure.

CMS restructured its deficiency code system beginning on November 28, 2017, and, due to these coding changes, we did not analyze CMS data cited by surveyors after the implementation of that change.

Percentages may not add to 100 due to rounding.

Figure 2. Severity of Cited Abuse Deficiencies, 2013 through 2017.

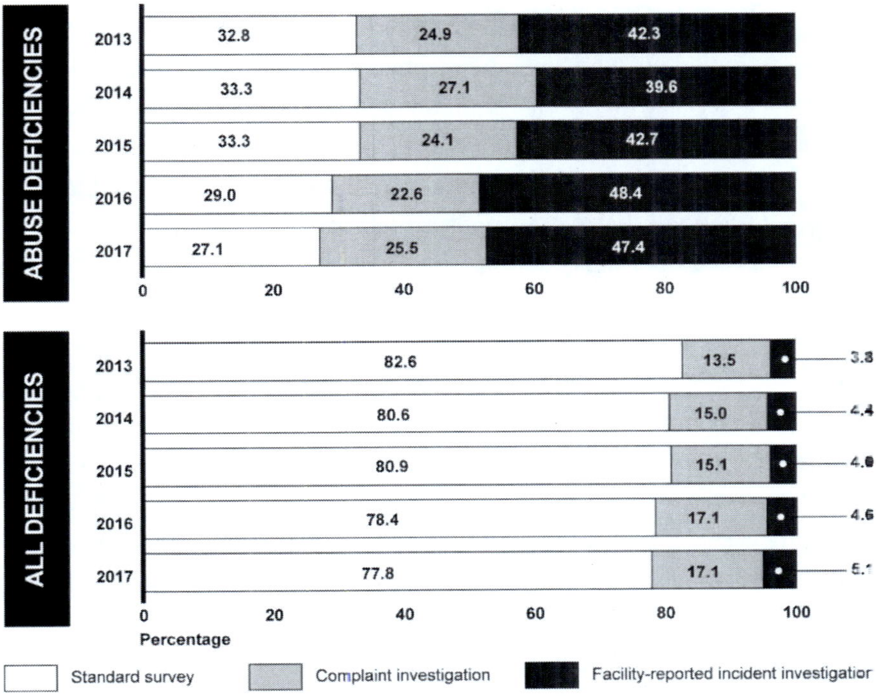

Source: GAO analysis of Centers for Medicare & Medicaid Services' (CMS) data. | GAO-19-433

Notes: For 375 out of 2,892 abuse deficiencies and 55,190 out of 538,559 total deficiencies cited over the 5-year time period, we were unable to determine from CMS's data whether the deficiency was identified during a standard survey, complaint investigation, facility-reported incident investigation, or a combination. We excluded these deficiencies from our percentages in the figure.

CMS restructured its deficiency code system beginning on November 28, 2017, and, due to these coding changes, we did not analyze CMS data cited by surveyors after the implementation of that change.

Percentages may not add to 100 due to rounding.

Figure 3. Type of Survey or Investigation Used to Identify Abuse Deficiencies and All Types of Deficiencies, 2013 through 2017.

We found that enforcement actions—or penalties—were imposed and implemented by CMS infrequently each year in response to abuse deficiencies, and that fines were the most common type of implemented penalty. Specifically, for each year from 2013 through 2017, we found that about one-third of abuse deficiencies had an enforcement action imposed but not implemented, and less than 8 percent of abuse deficiencies had enforcement actions that were implemented against the nursing home.[32] This was fairly consistent over the 5-year period.[33] For example, in 2017, of the 875 abuse deficiencies cited, 275 (31.4 percent) resulted in enforcement actions that were imposed but not implemented and 65 (7.4 percent) had enforcement actions that were implemented against the nursing home. Furthermore, for abuse deficiencies cited at the most severe levels—that is, those causing actual harm or immediate jeopardy to residents—a smaller percentage of the deficiencies had an enforcement action imposed but not implemented compared to all abuse deficiencies, but a larger percentage were implemented. For example, in 2017, 373 of the 875 abuse deficiencies were cited at the most severe levels; of those, 81 (21.7 percent) resulted in enforcement actions that were imposed but not implemented, and 51 (13.7 percent) were implemented against the nursing home. Regardless of the severity, the predominant reason that CMS did not implement imposed enforcement actions was because the nursing home came into compliance prior to the implementation date of the penalty.[34]

For implemented enforcement actions, fines—known as civil money penalties—were overwhelmingly the most common type of penalty implemented against nursing homes with abuse deficiencies, increasing from 69.6 percent of the 23 abuse deficiencies with implemented enforcement actions in 2013 to 83.1 percent of the 65 in 2017. Denial of payments for new Medicare and Medicaid admissions—another financial penalty—was the second most common type of implemented enforcement action, but decreased from 34.8 percent in 2013 to 13.8 percent in 2017.

---

[32] The remaining abuse deficiencies did not have an enforcement action imposed or implemented. CMS may impose or implement more than one enforcement action in response to a single deficiency.

[33] The percent of all deficiencies that had an enforcement action imposed was also consistent over time but at a lower rate than for abuse deficiencies—about 27 percent. Similarly, the percent of all deficiencies that ultimately resulted in an implemented penalty against the nursing home was less than for abuse deficiencies—staying at about 2 percent each year.

[34] Other reasons that an imposed enforcement action may not be implemented include the CMS regional office changing its decision, the state survey agency changing its recommendation, or that an informal dispute resolution removed the associated level of noncompliance, among others.

Mandatory termination is the most severe enforcement action as it ends all payments for Medicare and Medicaid residents; it is implemented very rarely, with only one abuse deficiency resulting in mandatory termination of the nursing home across all 5 years.[35] (See Figure 4.)

In addition, we found the number of nursing homes with abuse deficiencies also more than doubled over the 5-year period. In 2013, 394 nursing homes (2.7 percent of all surveyed nursing homes) had at least one abuse deficiency compared to 821 nursing homes (5.6 percent of all surveyed nursing homes) in 2017. A nursing home may have more than one abuse deficiency cited in a single year, such as from a standard survey early in the year and then a complaint investigation later in the year. We found that in 2013, of the 394 nursing homes that had a total of 430 abuse deficiencies cited, 85 of the homes had two or more abuse deficiencies that year. In 2017, of the 821 nursing homes that had 875 total abuse deficiencies cited, 155 had two or more that year.

Further, across the 5-year period, we found that a small proportion of all nursing homes with abuse deficiencies had them in multiple consecutive years. Specifically, across all years, 2,214 total unique nursing homes (13.6 percent of all surveyed nursing homes) had at least one abuse deficiency. A small portion of these nursing homes had at least one abuse deficiency in multiple consecutive years, indicating potential patterns in abuse at these nursing homes. Specifically, 185 of the 2,214 nursing homes with abuse deficiencies over the 5-year period—8.4 percent—had an abuse deficiency

---

[35] Over the 5 years, some abuse deficiencies resulted in other types of enforcement actions, such as directed in-service training (where the nursing home is required to provide training to staff on a specific issue) and state monitoring (where an on-site monitor is placed in the nursing home to help ensure that the home achieves and maintains compliance).
We found similar proportions and trends in the enforcement actions implemented against nursing homes with any type of deficiency. For instance, civil money penalties were also the most commonly implemented enforcement action and increased from 61.5 percent of implemented actions in 2013 to 76.8 percent in 2017. Denial of payment for new Medicare and Medicaid admissions was also the second most common action implemented and decreased from 23.3 percent in 2013 to 16.2 percent in 2017. Mandatory termination was also rare, with a total of 43 nursing homes terminated over the 5 years. In 2007, we also found that the majority of enforcement actions implemented from fiscal years 2000 through 2005 were civil money penalties. See GAO, *Nursing Homes: Efforts to Strengthen Federal Enforcement Have Not Deterred Some Homes from Repeatedly Harming Residents*, GAO-07-241 (Washington, D.C., Mar. 26, 2007).

in any 2 consecutive years. In addition, 25 of the nursing homes—1.1 percent—had an abuse deficiency in 3 or more consecutive years.[36] (See Figure 5.)

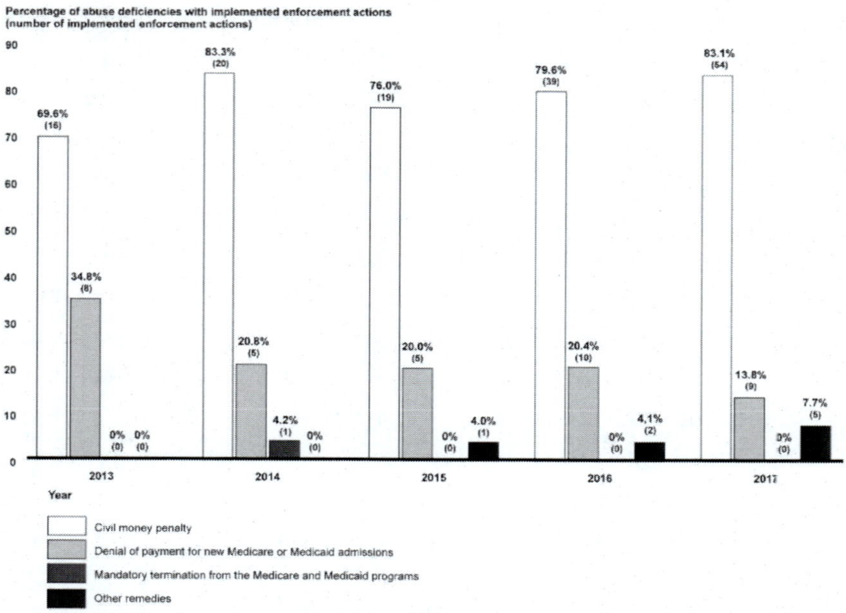

Source: GAO analysis of Centers for Medicare & Medicaid Services' (CMS) data. | GAO-19-433

Notes: Percentages do not add to 100 because a single deficiency may result in more than one enforcement action.

Other remedies include enforcement actions such as directed in-service training (where the nursing home is required to provide training to staff on a specific issue) and state monitoring (where an on- site monitor is placed in the nursing home to help ensure that the home achieves and maintains compliance).

CMS restructured its deficiency code system beginning on November 28, 2017 and, due to these coding changes, we did not analyze CMS data cited by surveyors after the implementation of that change.

Figure 4. Types of Implemented Enforcement Actions for Abuse Deficiencies, 2013 through 2017.

---

[36] An additional 143 nursing homes had an abuse deficiency in any 2 nonconsecutive years, and an additional 35 nursing homes had an abuse deficiency in any 3 or 4 nonconsecutive years, from 2013 through 2017.

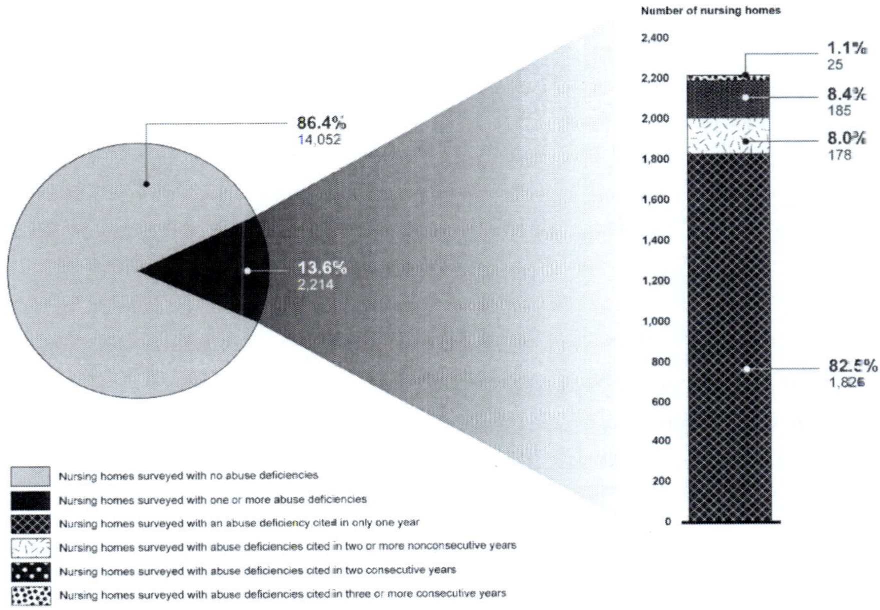

Source: GAO analysis of Centers for Medicare & Medicaid Services' (CMS) data. | GAO-19-433

Note: CMS restructured its deficiency code system beginning on November 28, 2017, and, due to these coding changes, we did not analyze CMS data cited by surveyors after the implementation of that change.

Figure 5. Nursing Homes with Abuse Deficiencies Cited in Multiple Years, 2013 through 2017.

Finally, we analyzed a selection of characteristics, including ownership type and bed size, for these nursing homes that had abuse deficiencies cited in multiple years and compared them to homes that had abuse deficiencies cited in a single year and surveyed homes that did not have any abuse deficiencies. We found that the nursing homes differed. For example while for-profit organizations—the largest ownership group accounting for 67.9 percent of all surveyed nursing homes—owned 66.9 percent of nursing homes without any abuse deficiencies cited over the 5-year period, they accounted for 78.6 percent of nursing homes that had abuse deficiencies cited in 2 or more years.[37] In addition, nursing homes designated as Special Focus Facilities—a CMS program that provides increased oversight to homes with consistent poor performance—constituted 2.5 percent of all surveyed nursing homes compared to 1.9 percent of nursing homes without abuse deficiencies and 10.1 percent of nursing homes with abuse deficiencies cited in 2 or more years.[38] (See Table 2.)

Physical and Mental/Verbal Abuse Occurred Most Often, Followed by Sexual Abuse, and Staff Were More Often Perpetrators of Abuse in 2016 and 2017

Our analysis of a representative sample of CMS narrative descriptions—written by state surveyors—associated with abuse deficiencies cited in 2016 and 2017 found that physical and mental/verbal abuse occurred most often in nursing homes, followed by sexual abuse. Further, staff were more often the perpetrators of the deficiencies cited as abuse than were residents or others.[39] (See Figure 6.)

---

[37] These results are consistent with our analyses in both a 2009 and 2016 report. In those reports, we determined the number of nursing homes with consistent poor quality performance over time and found that they were also more likely to be for-profit or large homes with more than 100 beds compared to homes that performed well. However, our methodologies for each analysis vary. See GAO, *Nursing Homes: CMS's Special Focus Facility Methodology Should Better Target the Most Poorly Performing Homes, Which Tended to Be Chain Affiliated and For-Profit*. GAO-09-689 (Washington, D.C.: Aug. 28, 2009) and GAO-16-33.

[38] Nursing homes with chronic noncompliance with federal standards can be selected for the Special Focus Facility program, which requires state survey agencies to conduct more frequent oversight and the nursing homes to improve performance or risk termination from the Medicare and Medicaid programs. For more information on this program, see GAO, *Poorly Performing Nursing Homes: Special Focus Facilities Are Often Improving, but CMS's Program Could Be Strengthened*, GAO-10-197 (Washington, D.C.: Mar. 19, 2010).

[39] Because abuse and perpetrator type are not readily identifiable in the CMS data, we identified this information by reviewing a representative sample of the narratives written by surveyors from 2016 through 2017 that describe substantiated abuse. Percentages may not add to 100 because some narratives had multiple types of abuse; some described involuntary seclusion, which was included in CMS's abuse deficiency code during the time period we examined; some deficiencies had narratives that were missing or incomplete; and some narratives described deficiencies that were not consistent with CMS's definition of abuse—for example, neglect or misappropriation.

Table 2. Characteristics of Nursing Homes with Multiple Years of Abuse Deficiencies, a Single Year of Abuse Deficiencies, or No Abuse Deficiencies, 2013 through 2017

	Nursing homes with an abuse deficiency in 2 or more years	Nursing homes with an abuse deficiency in a single year	Nursing homes without any abuse deficiencies	All surveyed nursing homes
Type of ownership				
For-profit	78.6%	73.0%	66.9%	67.9%
Nonprofit	13.9%	17.7%	24.5%	23.5%
Government-owned	5.2%	6.1%	6.0%	6.0%
Mixed ownership[a]	1.3%	2.0%	1.1%	1.2%
Location				
Urban	76.3%	69.1%	68.1%	68.4%
Rural	19.6%	27.1%	27.8%	27.5%
Transitioning area[b]	3.1%	2.7%	2.8%	2.8%
Number of Medicare and Medicaid certified beds				
Small (Less than 50)	3.9%	7.2%	14.0%	13.0%
Medium (50 to 99)	35.1%	38.0%	36.3%	36.5%
Large (100 to 199)	49.7%	47.6%	42.6%	43.4%
Very large (200 or more)	11.3%	7.2%	7.0%	7.1%
Special Focus Facility program				
Participated in program	10.1%	4.9%	1.9%	2.5%
Average Five-Star System overall quality rating[c]				
1 star	16.8%	11.0%	4.5%	5.5%
2 stars	44.1%	32.4%	19.1%	21.2%
3 stars	22.2%	28.8%	25.9%	26.1%
4 stars	12.4%	19.8%	29.7%	28.1%
5 stars	3.6%	6.8%	19.0%	17.3%

Source: GAO analysis of Centers for Medicare & Medicaid Services' data. | GAO-19-433.

Notes: Percentages do not always add to 100 due to missing data and rounding. The percentage of nursing homes with missing data was less than 2 percent for each category.

CMS restructured its deficiency code system beginning on November 28, 2017, and, due to these coding changes, we did not analyze CMS data cited by surveyors after the implementation of that change.

[a] "Mixed ownership" refers to nursing homes that changed their profit status at any point over the five-year period.

[b] A "transitioning area" is where the designation changed from rural to urban or vice-versa at some point during the five-year period.

[c] The Five-Star Quality Rating System assigns nursing homes with an overall "star" rating, ranging from one to five. Nursing homes with five stars are considered to have much above average quality, while nursing homes receiving one star are considered to have much below average quality.

- Physical abuse, which CMS defines as hitting, slapping, punching, biting and kicking residents, was present in about 46 percent (+/- 5 percent) of the abuse deficiency narratives.
- Mental/verbal abuse, which CMS defines as verbal or nonverbal conduct that can cause a resident to experience humiliation and fear, among other things, was present in about 44 percent (+/- 5 percent) of the abuse deficiency narratives.
- Sexual abuse, which CMS defines as non-consensual sexual contact with a resident, was present in about 18 percent (+/- 5 percent) of the abuse deficiency narratives.[40]

Staff, which includes those working in any part of the nursing home, were perpetrators in 58 percent (+/- 5 percent) of abuse deficiency narratives, followed by resident perpetrators (30 percent +/- 5 percent) and other types of perpetrators (2 percent +/- 5 percent).[41] Other types of perpetrators can include family members of residents or other visitors.

Further, our analysis of the narratives found that sexual abuse perpetrated by residents (39 percent) occurred more frequently within our sample than sexual abuse perpetrated by staff (10 percent) or others (17 percent).[42] When staff were the perpetrators of abuse, we found within our sample that mental/verbal abuse was the most common type of abuse (60 percent), while physical abuse was most common in situations where residents (59 percent) or others (67 percent) were the perpetrators. For examples of the different types of abuse and perpetrators from our analysis, see Table 3 below. Within our sample of narratives, mental/verbal abuse was less likely to be categorized by surveyors as severe compared to physical and sexual abuse.

---

[40] Upper and lower confidence levels were: physical (41 to 51 percent), mental/verbal (40 to 49 percent), and sexual abuse (14 to 22 percent).

[41] Upper and lower confidence levels were: staff-on-resident (54 to 63 percent), resident- on-resident (26 to 35 percent), and other (1 to 3 percent).

[42] Information in this paragraph describes our sample but is not representative of all abuse deficiency narratives.

Table 3. Examples from a Representative Sample of Nursing Home Abuse Deficiency Narratives, 2016-2017

Type(s) of abuse	Type(s) of perpetrator	Narrative details	Scope and severity
Physical abuse	Staff	A nurse aide grabbed a resident by both wrists, causing the resident to fall to the floor and resulting in bruising to the resident's left wrist and left hip.	Isolated scope, immediate jeopardy
Physical and sexual abuse	Resident	Resident 1, who had severe cognitive impairment, kicked another Resident 2, who also had significant cognitive impairment, in the face. Separately, Resident 3 shoved Resident 4 against a door, causing Resident 4 to fall. After being helped up by staff, Resident 4 was hit by Resident 3. The same resident (Resident 3) later slapped a different resident—Resident 5 in the head. Also in the narrative, Resident 6 fondled the breast of Resident 7, who appeared confused by the action.	Isolated scope, actual harm
Sexual and mental/verbal abuse	Resident and staff	A cognitively impaired resident (Resident 1) with a history of inappropriate sexual behavior grabbed Resident 2 in a sexually inappropriate manner. Resident 1 then grabbed the "private area" of Resident 3. Separately, a nursing home dietary staff member was verbally abusive to a resident (Resident 4), yelling and antagonizing the resident.	Widespread, immediate jeopardy
Sexual abuse	Staff	A nurse aide found a medical technician sexually assaulting a resident in the resident's room. The resident was non-verbal, with severe dementia, and was totally dependent on staff for mobility. The medical technician "begged" the nursing assistant not to tell anyone about witnessing the assault, and the medical technician later told a supervisor they had had "this problem for a while."	Isolated scope, immediate jeopardy
Mental/verbal abuse	Other	Resident 1 had an argument with Resident 2. Resident 2's family member arrived and threatened to kick Resident 1 out of her wheelchair if she did not stay away from Resident 2. Resident 1 was deeply concerned and felt frightened every time Resident 2's family member visited and she said that she had a nightmare about the family member.	Isolated scope, no actual harm with a potential for more than minimal harm
Mental/verbal abuse	Staff	A nurse assistant told a resident to "shut up and (expletive) off" when the resident requested to have their soiled brief changed, and the facility staff member put the resident's call light on the floor under the resident's bed so that the resident would not turn on the call light when they needed care. The state survey agency investigated this complaint, which had not been reported to the facility administrator.	Isolated scope, actual harm

Source: GAO summary of Centers for Medicare & Medicaid Services' (CMS) data. | GAO-19-433.

Notes: We reviewed a representative sample of abuse deficiency narratives from CMS to determine the most common abuse type and perpetrator type.

Specifically, we found in our sample that the proportion of mental/verbal abuse (30 percent) categorized by state surveyors as severe—defined as actual harm or immediate jeopardy—was smaller than the proportion of physical (40 percent) and sexual abuse (58 percent) categorized as severe. In addition, we found that most of the mental/verbal (88 percent), physical (91 percent), and sexual abuse (77 percent) narratives in our sample were categorized by surveyors as "isolated" in scope.[43]

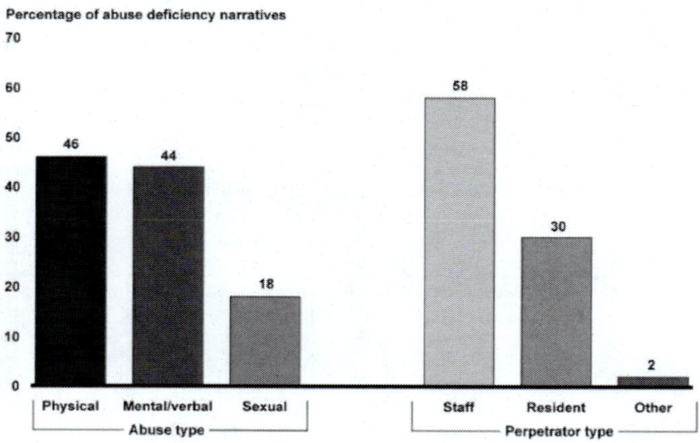

Source: GAO analysis of Centers for Medicare & Medicaid Services' (CMS) data and supporting narratives. | GAO-19-433

Notes: We reviewed a representative sample of abuse deficiency narratives from CMS to determine the most common abuse type and perpetrator type. Percentages do not add to 100 because some narratives had multiple types of abuse, some deficiencies had narratives that were missing or incomplete, and some narratives described deficiencies that were not consistent with CMS's definition of abuse—for example, neglect or misappropriation. In addition, CMS's abuse deficiency code also included involuntary seclusion in the time period we examined. Our analysis found that 3 percent of the abuse deficiency narratives were attributable to involuntary seclusion.

Figure 6. Representative Sample of Nursing Home Abuse Deficiency Narratives, by Abuse Type and Perpetrator Type, 2016 through 2017.

---

[43] The remaining narratives in our sample were categorized as: "pattern" (mental/verbal—11 percent, physical—8 percent, sexual—19 percent) and "widespread" (mental/verbal—1 percent, physical—1 percent, sexual—4 percent).

STAKEHOLDERS IDENTIFIED RESIDENT CHARACTERISTICS AND STAFFING INADEQUACIES AS RISK FACTORS FOR ABUSE, AND UNDERREPORTING AS AMONG THE CHALLENGES TO INVESTIGATING ABUSE

Some Resident Characteristics and Inadequacies in Staffing, Training, and Staff Screening Can Increase Risk of Abuse

Stakeholder groups in most of the five states we interviewed—including state survey agencies, Adult Protective Services, law enforcement, MFCUs, ombudsmen, and nursing home administrators and clinical staff—identified risk factors for abuse in nursing homes that included resident characteristics, such as residents with infrequent visitors, and nursing home staffing characteristics, such as insufficient staffing levels. (See Table 4 for a description of these risk factors.) Officials we interviewed from national organizations with knowledge of abuse in nursing homes also noted some of these same risk factors.

Table 4. Risk Factors for Nursing Home Abuse Identified by Stakeholders

Risk factor	Description
Resident characteristics	• Residents with cognitive impairment can be at an increased risk for abuse because they may have difficulty recalling recent events. • Residents with infrequent visitors can be at an increased risk for abuse because regular visitors can notice and report changes in behavior or physical appearance. • Elderly nursing home residents who are mixed with widely differing age groups, such as young adults with mental illness, can be at an increased risk for abuse.
Nursing home staffing characteristics	• Nursing homes with insufficient staff can lead to too few staff attending to the needs of residents and to staff feeling overworked—both of which can lead to abuse. • Nursing homes with inadequate staff training can be at risk for abuse because staff may not know how to diffuse challenging situations with residents or know how to identify and report abuse. • Nursing homes with inadequate staff screening, such as through background checks and the nurse aide registry, could result in hiring staff with histories of abuse.

Source: GAO stakeholder interviews. | GAO-19-433.

Note: We interviewed officials from stakeholder groups including state survey agencies, Adult Protective Services law enforcement, Medicaid Fraud Control Units, ombudsmen, and nursing homes.

Resident Characteristics

Stakeholders in each of our five selected states noted that residents who do not have frequent visitors, are cognitively impaired, or mixed with widely different age groups may be at an increased risk for abuse.

- Residents who do not have frequent visitors. Stakeholders in four of the five states said that residents without regular visitors, such as family, may be at an increased risk for abuse because regular visitors could notice and report potential warning signs of abuse, such as changes in their behavior or physical appearance.
- Residents who are cognitively impaired. Stakeholders in each of the five states said that cognitively impaired residents may be especially vulnerable to abuse because they often cannot speak or may have difficulty recalling recent events, and they are therefore less likely to be able to remember or describe what happened. In addition to noting that cognitively impaired residents may be at an increased risk of abuse, some stakeholders said that some cognitively impaired residents may be more likely to be perpetrators of abuse as their condition can have behavioral symptoms, such as physical aggressiveness.
- Residents mixed with widely different age groups. Stakeholders in four of the five states also noted that elderly nursing home residents who are mixed with widely differing age groups, such as young adults with mental illness, may be at a higher risk for incidents of abuse due to the different characteristics of these groups. Combining these two populations, which have differing needs, can also be challenging for staff. For example, staff may have more experience caring for elderly residents with complex needs, such as dementia, and they may not have the necessary skills or training to care for needs of younger residents, who require other types of complex care. This can create a stressful environment for staff, which is a risk factor for staff as potential perpetrators of abuse. Two stakeholders noted that younger residents who may have mental illness can have conflicts with

older and frailer residents, potentially leading to abusive incidents between residents.

Nursing Home Staffing Characteristics

Stakeholders we interviewed in each of our five selected states noted that nursing homes with insufficient staffing, inadequate staff training, and inadequate staff screening may be at risk for abuse.

- Nursing homes with insufficient staff. Stakeholders in each of the five states said that nursing homes with insufficient staff may be at risk for abuse because there may not be enough staff attending to the needs of residents.[44] Stakeholders noted that nursing homes have faced challenges hiring and retaining qualified staff and that, as a result, existing staff can feel overworked, stressed, or exhausted, which can lead to abusive behaviors. Staffing issues are not just risk factors for staff as perpetrators of abuse, but they can also limit a staff member's ability to identify and report abuse. For example, insufficient staffing may mean that there are not enough available staff to notice signs of abuse in a timely fashion, such as noticing a resident's bruises before they heal.
- Nursing homes with inadequate staff training on abuse. Inadequate staff training on abuse was noted by stakeholders we interviewed in four of the five states as a risk factor for abuse because; for example, staff may not know how to diffuse challenging situations

[44] Numerous studies have established a relationship between higher nurse staffing levels and better care outcomes in nursing homes. In 1996, the Institute of Medicine concluded that a preponderance of evidence demonstrates a positive relationship between nurse staffing and quality of care in nursing homes. Federal law does not require a minimum nurse staff to resident ratio. A 2001 CMS study recommended a minimum staffing ratio per resident; however, CMS has not implemented these recommendations. See Institute of Medicine, U.S. Committee on the Adequacy of Nursing Staff in Hospitals and Nursing Homes, G Wunderlick, F Sloan, CK Davis, *Nursing Staff in Hospitals and Nursing Homes: Is it Adequate?* (Washington, D.C.: National Academies Press, 1996). Also see Centers for Medicare & Medicaid Services, *Report to Congress: Appropriateness of Minimum Nurse Staffing Ratios in Nursing Homes, Phase II Final Report* (Baltimore, Md.: December 2001).

with residents and identify and report abuse.[45] As previously noted, recognizing abuse can be challenging and, even when abuse is identified, it is often not reported. Officials from all of the nursing homes that we visited said that they provide training to their staff on abuse, including on defining abuse, identifying or detecting different types of abuse, and reporting abuse.[46] Staff members we spoke with at one nursing home said that, not only are they trained to look for physical signs of abuse, such as bruising, but they are also trained to observe changes in behavior that may be warning signs for abuse, such as a resident suddenly withdrawing from group activities. Staff at another nursing home said that they are also taught to ask another staff member for assistance when they are feeling frustrated or stressed by caring for a particular resident. In contrast, staff at another nursing home noted the challenges of not having these types of resources and said they are needed at their facility.

- Nursing homes with inadequate staff screening. Stakeholders in three of our five states said that inadequate staff screening can be a risk factor for abuse. Some stakeholders said that a thorough background screening can be time consuming. Further, because staff screening through background checks and the nurse aide registry is not coordinated across the country, there are gaps that could enable individuals who committed crimes in one state to obtain employment at a nursing home in another state, a concern that we previously reported.[47] Staff from a nursing home we visited

---

[45] Federal law requires nursing homes to provide training for all new and existing staff on preventing, identifying, and reporting abuse. 42 C.F.R. § 483.95(c) (2018).

[46] Some stakeholders also noted that they have provided training to residents on, for example, understanding their rights and how to report abuse.

[47] CMS requires nursing homes to establish policies that prevent the hiring of individuals who have been convicted of abusing nursing home residents but does not require that they conduct background checks—either statewide or nationally. States, however, may require that background checks be conducted. States vary in terms of whether the background check must be statewide, national, or both, and in other requirements of these checks. A 2011 OIG report found that almost all nursing homes employed one or more individuals with at least one criminal conviction. See HHS OIG, *Nursing Facilities' Employment of Individuals with Criminal Convictions*. OEI-07-09-00110. (Washington, D.C.: March 2011). In 2010, the Affordable Care Act required the establishment of the National Background Check

said the prevention of abuse "starts with hiring the right staff" and noted the importance of conducting background checks and checking references for prospective employees.

Underreporting of Abuse, Cognitive Impairment of Victims, Lack of Nursing Home Cooperation, and Lack of Agency Coordination Pose Challenges for Abuse Investigations

The key challenges for abuse investigations most frequently identified by stakeholder groups in the five states we reviewed were underreporting of abuse, cognitive impairment of victims, lack of cooperation from nursing homes, and lack of agency coordination.[48] (See Table 5 for a description of these challenges.) Officials we interviewed from national organizations with knowledge of abuse in nursing homes also noted some of these same challenges.

Underreporting of Abuse

Stakeholders in each of the five states in our review noted that abuse in nursing homes may be underreported because residents or their families feel uncomfortable or fear retaliation from nursing home staff.[49] For

---

Program, which provides grants to states to design national comprehensive background check programs for long term care facility and provider employees. As of February 2019, CMS officials told us that there have been 29 states in the National Background Check program and 11 of these states are still active. CMS also requires nursing homes to check the state nurse aide registry before hiring a prospective nurse aide to ensure there is not a finding of abuse. However, nurse aide registries only reflect an aide's history in a particular state. And although there are multi-state registry verification requirements, including that nursing homes seek information from every state registry in states where they believe the aide has worked, we and HHS OIG have raised concerns about state nurse aide registries, and OIG recommended that CMS seek legislative authority to create a national nurse aide registry. See GAO-02-312 and HHS OIG, *Nurse Aide Registries: State Compliance and Practices. OEI-07-03-00380.* (Washington, D.C.: February 2005). While the Elder Justice Act required HHS to conduct a study on the feasibility of establishing a national nurse aide registry, HHS officials reported that because Congress has not appropriated funding for this provision of the Act, the study has not been completed.

48 The stakeholders we interviewed included state survey agencies, Adult Protective Services, law enforcement, MFCUs, ombudsmen, and nursing homes.

49 This is consistent with findings from a National Research Council publication: C. Hawes, *Elder Abuse in Residential Long-Term Care Settings: What is Known and What Information*

example, residents who were sexually abused may feel ashamed or embarrassed to report these incidents. In addition, residents may fear retaliation by the nursing home staff on whom they depend, which might include substandard care, exclusion from activities, or even eviction from the home. A fear of retaliation can also extend to nursing home staff, who may witness abuse by another staff member, but may be afraid to report it out of fear that they will lose their jobs or that they will face retaliation from co-workers. This underreporting creates challenges for investigators, who are unable to investigate if they do not know that abuse has occurred.

Table 5. Key Challenges for Abuse Investigations Identified by Stakeholders

Key challenge	Description
Underreporting of abuse	Abuse in nursing homes may not be reported because residents or their family members may feel uncomfortable or fear retaliation from staff at the nursing home. In addition, nursing home staff may be afraid to report abuse out of fear of losing their jobs.
Cognitive impairment of victims	Residents with cognitive impairment may not recall the abuse that occurred, may not be able to verbalize a statement regarding the abuse, or may not be considered reliable witnesses.
Lack of cooperation from some nursing homes	Nursing homes may withhold, alter, or make it difficult for investigatory agencies to gain access to necessary, timely, or accurate information about alleged abuse.
Lack of agency coordination	Having multiple agencies involved in investigations can create challenges, such as coordinating investigations and notifying one another about investigation outcomes.

Source: GAO stakeholder interviews. | GAO-19-433.

Note: We interviewed officials from stakeholder groups including state survey agencies, Adult Protective Services, law enforcement, Medicaid Fraud Control Units, ombudsmen, and nursing homes.

Cognitive Impairment of Victims

Stakeholders in each of the five states in our review said that victims with cognitive impairment may not be able to give statements regarding the abuse or may not be considered reliable witnesses. For example, residents with dementia may not be able to remember the details of an abusive incident, and their memory of the details may deteriorate over the

---

is Needed? National Research Council of the National Academies. (Washington, D.C.: 2003).

course of an investigation. Or, residents with dementia may report abuse that stems from traumatic memories from an incident that occurred earlier in their lives. One stakeholder said this can be a challenge for investigations because they do not know how much they can rely on a cognitively impaired resident's statement, making it difficult for them to corroborate an abuse allegation. However, one stakeholder noted that, while it can be difficult to interview abuse victims with cognitive impairment, it is important to treat their allegations seriously and with credibility. One law enforcement stakeholder noted that interviews with these victims require special training.

Lack of Cooperation from Some Nursing Homes

Stakeholders in each of the five states in our review said that some nursing homes may withhold, alter, or make it difficult for investigatory agencies to gain access to necessary, timely, or accurate information about alleged abuse. This may be, for example, because they may fear adverse publicity, litigation, or penalties from the state or CMS. In addition, as noted previously, nursing home staff may be fearful of losing their jobs. Stakeholders said that nursing home staff who witnessed abuse may be intentionally vague when interviewed by investigators; for example, by saying they cannot recall an incident. Some stakeholders also noted that nursing homes may delay investigators' access to patient records, or they may even alter patient records in order to fill in information that should have been documented but was not at the time of the incident. One stakeholder we interviewed noted that the problem is not necessarily widespread—that some nursing homes are open about sharing information while others can be more difficult. Another stakeholder noted that a nursing home's cooperation can sometimes depend on the seriousness of the allegation.

Lack of Agency Coordination

Stakeholders in three of the five states in our review said that having multiple agencies involved in investigations, such as the state survey agency, law enforcement, the ombudsman, and, in some states, Adult

Protective Services, can create challenges, including coordinating investigations and notifying one another about investigation outcomes. One stakeholder said they sometimes begin an investigation without realizing another investigatory agency has already started its own investigation. Further, stakeholders in two of the five states in our review said that CMS does not allow state survey agencies to share important investigatory information with law enforcement. (We discuss this issue in more detail later in this report.)

CMS's Ability to Ensure Nursing Home Residents Are Free from Abuse May Be Limited by Gaps in Oversight

We found that CMS: (1) cannot readily access data on the type of abuse or type of perpetrator, (2) has not provided guidance on what information nursing homes should include in facility-reported incidents, and (3) has numerous gaps in its referral process that can result in delayed and missed referrals to other entities. Together, these gaps affect critical points in CMS's oversight of abuse in nursing homes including the prevention, identification, and timely investigation of abuse.

Information on Abuse and Perpetrator Types Is Not Readily Available

CMS cannot readily access information on abuse or perpetrator type in its datasets and, as a result, lacks key information critical to understanding and appropriately addressing nursing home abuse with its oversight. Specifically, in two of CMS's datasets—complaints/facility-reported incidents and deficiencies—agency officials told us they do not require the state survey agencies to record abuse and perpetrator type.[50] As a result, we

[50] While there is a field in the complaints/facility-reported incidents database that allows state survey agencies to record data on abuse type and perpetrator type, as of March 2019 CMS

found that CMS's data do not readily support CMS's understanding of the types of abuse and perpetrators that are most prevalent in nursing homes. CMS officials told us they believe that the majority of abuse is committed by nursing home residents, and that physical and sexual abuse were the most common types; officials said they based this current understanding of abuse and perpetrator types on professional experience, literature, and ad hoc analyses of deficiency narrative descriptions. However, our review of a representative sample of abuse deficiency narratives from 2016 and 2017 found that staff were more often the perpetrators of deficiencies cited as abuse than residents or others, and that physical and mental/verbal abuse occurred most often in nursing homes, followed by sexual abuse. CMS officials noted that some incidents resulting from resident altercations—particularly those that do not show a willful intent to harm—may not have been cited as an abuse deficiency by some state survey agencies and may have been cited as other deficiencies not specified as abuse. This may have contributed to the difference between CMS's understanding of the prevalence of resident to resident abuse and what their abuse deficiency data show.

If CMS required information on abuse and perpetrator type to be recorded, the agency would have a better understanding of abuse in nursing homes. However, CMS officials told us they do not currently require the state survey agencies to specify abuse and perpetrator type because they consider the surveyor's job to be identification and documentation of noncompliance.

---

officials told us that this field is optional for state survey agencies. We learned that two of the five state survey agencies in our review are recording and tracking data on abuse type and perpetrator type using this optional field in CMS's complaints/facility-reported incidents database. CMS officials told us that states can customize allegation sub-type for their internal use, and that, while its complaint/facility-reported incidents database does not capture perpetrator type data, states can customize the database to include optional data like alleged perpetrator type. CMS officials told us allegation sub-type data and data about alleged perpetrator type are not uploaded to national systems.

In the deficiency database, the narrative text associated with the deficiencies provides details on the incident, including information on the abuse type and perpetrator type. However, because these data are in an open text field format, they cannot be easily and accurately analyzed by the agency. Further, CMS officials told us they had not analyzed the abuse narratives.

Additionally, CMS officials told us they have not conducted a systematic review to gather information on abuse and perpetrator type. This is inconsistent with federal internal control standards directing management to use quality information to achieve program objectives.[51] Without the systematic collection and monitoring of specific abuse and perpetrator data, CMS lacks key information and, therefore, cannot take actions—such as tailoring prevention and investigation activities—to address the most prevalent types of abuse or perpetrators.

Facility-Reported Incidents Lack Key Information

All of the state survey agencies we spoke to told us that facility-reported incidents can lack key information that can cause potential delays in abuse investigations. Specifically, officials from each of the five state survey agencies told us that the facility-reported incidents they receive from nursing homes can lack key information that affects their ability to effectively triage incidents and determine whether an investigation should occur and how soon.[52] Two state survey agencies we spoke with said they sometimes have to conduct significant follow-up with the nursing homes to obtain the information they need to prioritize the incident for investigation—follow-up that delays and potentially negatively affects investigations.[53] For example, one state survey agency told us that a facility reported abuse involving two residents but did not initially report that the residents were injured, and that the facility did not file an addendum to the facility-reported incident to indicate resident injury.

---

[51] GAO-14-704G.

[52] Facility incident reports differ by state in the information requested and the method of delivery—for example, by online submission or by fax. These reports are filled out by facility staff and submitted to the state survey agency, which uses them to triage incident investigations.

[53] According to CMS, an unintended effect of the state survey agency calling the facility to gather additional information is that this can tip off nursing homes to a state survey agency investigation. Alerting a nursing home to an impending investigation could result in it changing the conditions that are typically present—for example, by altering evidence or changing documentation.

As a result of this incomplete information, the state survey agency did not properly prioritize this incident response.

Despite federal law requiring nursing homes to self-report allegations of abuse, and covered individuals to report reasonable suspicions of crimes against residents, CMS has not provided guidance on what information should be included in these reports. Our review of CMS's State Operations Manual found that CMS does not have guidance related to the information that nursing homes or covered individuals should report to the state survey agencies or local law enforcement; in contrast, it does contain guidance on the type of information members of the public should include in a complaint about nursing home quality to the state survey agency—and CMS makes a standardized complaint template form available on its website.[54]

The lack of guidance on the information that state survey agencies should collect on facility-reported incidents is inconsistent with federal internal control standards directing management to use quality information to achieve program objectives.[55] CMS could outline basic information requirements that states must include on incident forms used by nursing homes and covered individuals to ensure the state survey agency is receiving the information it needs to accurately and quickly triage these incidents. CMS officials told us in November 2018 that they have efforts underway to examine guidance related to the information state survey agencies need to appropriately triage these facility-reported incidents and are developing a facility-reported incident template. Until the guidance and template are in place, these facility-reported incidents may lack key information that can cause potential delays in abuse investigations.

---

[54] When we spoke to CMS officials in November 2018, they told us they recognize the need to provide more guidance on what information should be contained in facility incident reports, and that it is under development. However, they did not have a timeline available for implementation.

[55] GAO-14-704G.

Gaps Exist in CMS Process for State Survey Agency Referrals to Law Enforcement and MFCUs

CMS requires state survey agencies to make referrals to law enforcement and, if appropriate, to MFCUs when abuse is substantiated; however, we found numerous gaps in CMS's referral process that can result in delayed and missed referrals. (See Table 6.)

Table 6. Key Gaps in Centers for Medicare and Medicaid Services' (CMS) Process for Referrals

Gap in process	Description
Timing of abuse referrals	CMS requires state survey agencies to report abuse to law enforcement and Medicaid Fraud Control Units (MFCU), if appropriate, only after the abuse has been substantiated; as a result, investigations can be delayed.
Tracking of abuse referrals	CMS does not conduct oversight to ensure that state survey agency referrals to law enforcement and the MFCUs are occurring as required and may be missing non- compliance from the state survey agencies.
Definition of substantiated abuse	CMS's definition of substantiating an allegation is confusing to some state survey agencies, resulting in discrepancies in how state survey agencies interpret it and the potential that substantiated deficiencies would go unreported and not referred to law enforcement or MFCUs.
Information sharing with law enforcement	CMS's guidance on state survey agency referrals to law enforcement does not specify what information can be shared and may result in confusion or frustration for both state survey and law enforcement agencies and, ultimately, in delays in investigations.

Source: GAO analysis of information from CMS and state officials. | GAO-19-433.

Timing of Abuse Referrals

We found CMS's requirements for when state survey agencies should report abuse to law enforcement and MFCUs lag behind the federal requirements for when covered individuals should make such referrals, and, as a result, referrals may be significantly delayed. Specifically, federal law requires covered individuals to immediately report reasonable suspicions of a crime against a resident that results in serious bodily injury to law enforcement and the state survey agency.[56] Conversely, state survey agencies do not have to report suspicions of crime identified on complaints submitted to, and surveys conducted by, the state survey agency until the abuse has been substantiated—a process that can often take weeks or months.[57] Officials from one law enforcement agency and two MFCUs that we interviewed told us the delay in receiving referrals limits their ability to collect evidence and prosecute cases—for example, bedding associated with potential sexual abuse may have been washed and wounds may have healed. This is consistent with the findings of our 2002 report, where we recommended that CMS should ensure that state survey agencies immediately notify law enforcement or MFCUs when nursing homes report allegations of physical or sexual abuse.[58] One state survey agency in our review established more stringent guidelines than CMS by requiring the surveyors to notify law enforcement and the MFCU promptly upon receiving a complaint of abuse. CMS officials told us their state survey agency reporting requirements are based on a March 2002 policy. This is inconsistent with standards for internal control, which state that management should communicate quality information externally so that external parties can help the entity achieve its objectives.[59]

---

[56] 42 U.S.C. § 1320b-25(b). These covered individuals include nursing home owners, operators, and employees, among others.

[57] CMS guidelines require referrals to law enforcement only after a finding of abuse is substantiated and referrals to MFCUs after substantiation "when appropriate," without clearly defining when a MFCU referral is warranted.

[58] CMS did not implement this recommendation from our 2002 report: it was closed as not implemented. GAO-02-312.
We also found delays in the amount of time it takes state survey agencies to make referrals to the nurse aide registry, potentially leaving nursing home residents at risk, and we recommended the time frame for determining whether to include findings of abuse in nurse aide registry files be shortened. (CMS did not implement this recommendation). This is also consistent with findings from an HHS OIG report. See Daniel R. Levinson, OIG, HHS, memorandum to Seema Verma, Administrator, CMS, *Early Alert: The Centers for Medicare & Medicaid Services Has Inadequate Procedures To Ensure That Incidents of Potential Abuse or Neglect at Skilled Nursing Facilities Are Identified and Reported in Accordance With Applicable Requirements*, A-01-17-00504 (Aug. 24, 2017).

[59] GAO-14-704G.

Tracking of Abuse Referrals

In addition to delays in referring cases to law enforcement and MFCUs, CMS officials also told us that CMS does not conduct oversight to ensure that state survey agency referrals to law enforcement and the MFCUs are occurring as required for substantiated abuse, and, as a result, CMS cannot ensure that state survey agencies are complying with reporting obligations. For example, an official from one of the five state survey agencies we interviewed said they had never made a referral to law enforcement or the MFCU, despite having substantiated allegations of abuse. The state survey agency official told us that they do not refer cases to law enforcement, and that law enforcement referrals are the responsibility of the nursing home. This is incompatible with CMS guidelines requiring that substantiated abuse be referred to law enforcement; however, CMS officials told us that they do not track whether state survey agencies make referrals to law enforcement and the MFCUs. This is inconsistent with federal standards for internal control, which state that management should establish and operate monitoring activities to monitor the internal control system and evaluate the results.[60]

Definition of Substantiated Abuse

We found confusion among some state survey agencies about CMS's definition of what it means to substantiate an allegation of abuse—a challenge because substantiation is a trigger in the investigation process, and CMS requires state survey agencies to make referrals to law enforcement and staff registries when abuse is substantiated by evidence. As a result, there is a potential for substantiated abuse to not be reported and, subsequently, not referred to law enforcement or MFCUs for criminal investigation. Two of the five state survey agencies in our review told us they believed they could not substantiate an allegation unless they could also cite a federal deficiency. This is inconsistent with CMS's guidance, which says that state survey agencies can substantiate that an allegation occurred without citing a federal deficiency and that, subsequently, these

---

[60] GAO-14-704G.

substantiated allegations must be referred to law enforcement and staff registries.[61] For example, according to CMS guidance, if the state survey agency investigated and found evidence that a resident was abused, but the nursing home had taken preventive actions against the deficient practice, the state survey agency would then substantiate that the abuse occurred, but not cite a deficiency. However, state survey agencies may decide not to substantiate an abuse allegation verified by evidence if they believe no deficiency should be cited, such as if the nursing home had taken preventive action against the deficient practice, which could result in that abuse going unreported and not referred to law enforcement, MFCUs, or staff registries. Because substantiation of abuse is a critical trigger in abuse investigations, confusion around its interpretation could prevent these important next steps.[62] CMS officials told us they are aware that the state survey agencies have varying interpretations of what it means to substantiate abuse. According to federal standards for internal control, management should internally communicate quality information to achieve the entity's objectives.[63]

Information Sharing

We also found that CMS's guidance on state survey agency referrals contained in its State Operations Manual does not specify what incident information can be shared with local law enforcement, either in response to local law enforcement's request for information or when the state survey agency refers substantiated findings of abuse to local law enforcement.[64] As a result, both state survey and law enforcement agencies expressed confusion and frustration about what information can be shared and said

---

[61] The other three state survey agencies we interviewed told us that they substantiate allegations without necessarily citing a federal deficiency, depending on the circumstances, as provided for in CMS guidance.

[62] We noted similar findings in a previous report, see GAO-11-280. In that report, we recommended that CMS clarify guidance to states about how particular fields in the database should be interpreted, such as what it means to substantiate a complaint. CMS has not implemented this recommendation.

[63] GAO-14-704G.

[64] State survey agencies are required to report substantiated findings of abuse to local law enforcement and MFCUs, if appropriate. State Operations Manual, Complaint Procedures, § 5330, Revision 155, June 10, 2016, CMS.

delays have occurred that can impede law enforcement investigations. Officials from two state survey agencies told us that CMS does not allow them to share any information with law enforcement without a written request.[65] For example, officials from one state survey agency said that they cannot share the name of the resident abused or the time when the incident occurred. One state survey agency said that information sharing can be uneven, and told us that law enforcement is required to share information with the state survey agencies, but the state survey agencies do not share their investigatory information with law enforcement. Officials from another state survey agency wrote to CMS notifying CMS of a change in their state survey agency protocol that would make the referral process timelier by providing un-redacted survey records of substantiated abuse to local law enforcement. However, in CMS's 2017 written response to the survey agency, CMS told them that all written requests for these records must continue to be forwarded to CMS for processing in accordance with the federal Privacy Act.

When we asked CMS officials what information state survey agencies can share with law enforcement in a referral, CMS explained that scenarios for requesting information can vary, and that CMS does not prescribe a specific method as it depends on the needs of the investigation. This lack of guidance is inconsistent with federal standards for internal control, which state that management should internally communicate quality information to achieve the entity's objectives.[66]

CONCLUSION

While nursing home abuse is relatively rare, our review shows that abuse deficiencies cited in nursing homes are becoming more frequent,

---

[65] HHS regulations implementing the Privacy Act provide that disclosure of information to another governmental entity is permitted "for a civil or criminal law enforcement activity if the activity is authorized by law, and if the head of such [governmental entity] has submitted a written request to the Department [of Health and Human Services] specifying the record desired and the law enforcement activity for which the record is sought." 45 C.F.R. § 5b.9(b)(7) (2018).

[66] GAO-14-704G.

with the largest increase in severe cases. As such, it is imperative that CMS have key information critical to understanding abuse and that the agency's oversight of nursing homes is strong. We found weaknesses in both CMS's understanding of abuse and in its oversight that need to be addressed. Specifically, because CMS cannot readily access information on abuse or perpetrator types in its data, it lacks key information critical to taking appropriate actions to address the most prevalent types of abuse and perpetrators. In addition, CMS has not provided guidance on what information should be included in facility-reported incidents, contributing to a lack of information for state survey agencies and, subsequently, delays in their investigations. This lack of guidance related to facility- reported incidents is important in light of our findings that abuse deficiencies are identified most commonly through facility-reported incidents. We also found other gaps in CMS's process related to ensuring timely referrals of abuse to law enforcement, tracking abuse referrals, defining abuse substantiation, and sharing information with law enforcement. These gaps affect CMS's oversight of abuse in nursing homes—including the prevention, identification and timely investigation of abuse—and may limit CMS's ability to ensure that nursing homes meet federal requirements for residents to be free from abuse.

RECOMMENDATIONS FOR EXECUTIVE ACTION

We are making the following six recommendations to the administrator of CMS:

Require that abuse and perpetrator type be submitted by state survey agencies in CMS's databases for deficiency, complaint, and facility-reported incident data, and that CMS systematically assess trends in these data. (Recommendation 1)

Develop and disseminate guidance—including a standardized form—to all state survey agencies on the information nursing homes and covered individuals should include on facility-reported incidents. (Recommendation 2)

Require state survey agencies to immediately refer complaints and surveys to law enforcement (and, when applicable, to MFCUs) if they have a reasonable suspicion that a crime against a resident has occurred when the complaint is received. (Recommendation 3)

Conduct oversight of state survey agencies to ensure referrals of complaints, surveys, and substantiated incidents with reasonable suspicion of a crime are referred to law enforcement (and, when applicable, to MFCUs) in a timely fashion. (Recommendation 4)

Develop guidance for state survey agencies clarifying that allegations verified by evidence should be substantiated and reported to law enforcement and state registries in cases where citing a federal deficiency may not be appropriate. (Recommendation 5)

Provide guidance on what information should be contained in the referral of abuse allegations to law enforcement. (Recommendation 6)

AGENCY COMMENTS

We provided a draft of this product to HHS for review and comment. In its comments, reproduced in appendix IV, HHS concurred with our six recommendations and identified actions it is taking to implement them. Specifically, HHS said that it will: (1) look into options for requiring state survey agencies to record data on abuse and perpetrator type so that HHS may assess trends in these data; (2) develop guidance that includes a list of standardized data elements to be included when nursing homes report facility-reported incidents and guidance specific to the reporting and tracking of facility-reported incidents involving abuse; (3) require state survey agencies to immediately refer complaints to law enforcement if a reasonable suspicion of a crime against a resident has occurred and share relevant survey information; (4) consider how to implement mechanisms for tracking law enforcement referrals; (5) identify opportunities to clarify in guidance situations where citing a federal deficiency may not be appropriate, but reporting the abuse is still required; and (6) develop a list of standardized elements that should be included when reporting an abuse allegation to law enforcement. HHS also provided technical comments, which we incorporated as appropriate.

As agreed with your offices, unless you publicly announce the contents of this report earlier, we plan no further distribution until 30 days from the report date. At that time, we will send copies to the Secretary of HHS and other interested parties.

John E. Dicken
Director, Health Care

APPENDIX I: ADDITIONAL DETAIL ON ANALYSIS OF CENTERS FOR MEDICARE & MEDICAID SERVICES' (CMS) DATA

This appendix describes our scope and methodology for determining the trends and types of abuse occurring in nursing homes in recent years. For this examination, we reviewed CMS guidance and analyzed data from 2013 through 2017, which represented the most recent data for a 5-year period at the time of our review. Specifically, we first reviewed the CMS State Operations Manual's Appendix PP that was in effect during our period of review to determine which federal standards and deficiency codes were relevant to resident abuse.[67] We focused our analysis on the deficiency code to be used by state surveyors when a nursing home fails to keep a resident free from abuse, which encompasses mental/verbal, sexual,

[67] Specifically, we reviewed Appendix PP of the State Operations Manual because it is the section that provides guidance to state surveyors about determining compliance with federal quality standards and their associated deficiency codes. There were multiple updates to Appendix PP of the State Operations Manual during the period of our review (January 1, 2013, through November 27, 2017). Specifically, there were eight updates to the appendix during the 5-year period, but none of these changed the abuse deficiency citation codes used by state surveyors. Therefore, we used the March 8, 2017, version of the Appendix PP—the most recent version during our period of review—when determining which deficiency codes to analyze for this report. CMS, *State Operations Manual, Appendix PP—Guidance to Surveyors for Long Term Care Facilities.* (March 8, 2017).
CMS restructured its deficiency code system beginning on November 28, 2017, and, due to these coding changes, we did not analyze CMS deficiency data cited by surveyors after the implementation of that change.

or physical abuse.[68] Surveyors can also use other deficiency codes for abuse-related issues, such as a failure by the nursing home to train staff on issues related to abuse, either in conjunction with an abuse deficiency or without an abuse deficiency. Since these abuse-related deficiency codes do not necessarily represent incidents of abuse, but do represent situations where a nursing home's inadequate policies could leave residents vulnerable to abuse, we conducted a limited analysis on the trends of these deficiencies, which is described in appendix II.

For our analysis, we identified abuse deficiencies cited by surveyors in all 50 states and Washington, D.C., between 2013 and 2017, using data provided by CMS from its Certification and Survey Provider Enhanced Reports system. Specifically, we calculated the number of abuse deficiencies cited each year and determined how many of these abuse deficiencies were at each level of severity—no actual harm with a potential for minimal harm, no actual harm with a potential for more than minimal harm, actual harm, and immediate jeopardy—for each year. We compared the results for abuse deficiencies with the results for all types of deficiencies in each year. To avoid over-counting deficiencies, deficiencies that were for the same violation on the same day for the same facility were counted as a single deficiency.[69] We then tracked (1) the origin of these abuse deficiencies and (2) enforcement actions implemented against nursing homes with these abuse deficiencies.

- Origin of abuse deficiencies. To identify trends in the origin of those abuse deficiencies—that is, whether the deficiency originated from a standard survey, complaint investigation, or a facility-reported incident investigation—we analyzed data

[68] For the purposes of this report, we refer to mental and verbal abuse as "mental/verbal abuse." Over the period of time examined in our review, CMS's abuse deficiency code also included involuntary seclusion.

[69] There are instances where a complaint is filed and the complaint investigation window coincides with a scheduled standard survey. CMS data records the deficiency as two separate records—as the result of a standard survey and as the result of a complaint investigation. Following CMS procedure, we counted this deficiency only once; however, we flagged that the deficiency resulted from a complaint and a standard survey. Consequently, the sum of the source of the deficiencies (complaint, facility-reported incident, and standard survey) will be greater than the number of deficiencies.

provided by CMS from its Automated Survey Processing Environment Complaint/Incident Tracking System. Specifically, we matched the deficiencies with the complaint/incident data using provider number, survey date, and deficiency code. We found that some deficiencies were the result of a combination of complaints, facility-reported incidents, surveys, or all three. We counted those deficiencies as originating from each relevant category.

- Enforcement actions. To identify trends in the enforcement actions imposed and implemented against nursing homes with abuse deficiencies, we analyzed data provided by CMS from its Automated Survey Processing Environment Enforcement Manager. Specifically, we matched the deficiencies with the enforcement data using provider number, survey date, case identification number, and deficiency code. To avoid over-counting, deficiencies that share the same code and case identification number were counted as a single deficiency. For each year, we determined how many of the abuse deficiencies resulted in enforcement actions imposed or implemented, the severity of the abuse deficiencies with enforcement actions, and the types of enforcement actions implemented.

We then examined these abuse deficiencies to determine the number of nursing homes that had abuse deficiencies, as well as the number of homes with repeated abuse deficiencies cited across the 5 years and the characteristics of those homes. We also determined the proportion of surveyed nursing homes in a given year that had an abuse deficiency.[70]

- Nursing homes that had repeated abuse deficiencies. Since a nursing home can have more than one abuse deficiency cited in a given year, we determined the number of surveyed nursing homes

[70] To determine the universe of nursing homes, we used the publicly available Nursing Home Compare Provider Information files to identify homes that had standard surveys with no deficiencies each year and combined those homes with homes that had deficiencies resulting from either standard surveys or investigations in data provided by CMS from its Certification and Survey Provider Enhanced Reports system.

each year that had at least one abuse deficiency, both nationally and by state. For each of those nursing homes, we determined if the home had an abuse deficiency repeated in multiple years and in two or more consecutive years.

- Nursing home characteristics. We attempted to identify commonalities among homes with multiple years of abuse deficiencies, homes with only a single year with an abuse deficiency, and surveyed homes without any abuse deficiencies throughout the 5-year period. Specifically, we matched deficiency data to CMS's publicly available Provider of Services files and the Nursing Home Compare Provider Information files for each nursing home; and we examined bed size, non-profit or for-profit status, Five-Star Quality Rating System overall rating, Special Focus Facility designation, and urban or rural location.[71]

Finally, because abuse and perpetrator type are not readily identifiable in CMS's data, we identified this information by reviewing the narratives written by surveyors that describe the substantiated abuse. Specifically, we obtained 1,557 narrative descriptions written by state surveyors for abuse deficiencies cited in 2016 and 2017 provided by CMS from its Automated Survey Processing Environment database.[72] From that universe of abuse deficiency narratives, we selected a randomly selected representative

---

[71] The CMS Provider of Services files were accessed on Dec. 14, 2018, from https:// www.cms.gov/Research-Statistics-Data-and-Systems/Downloadable-Public-Use- Files/ Provider-of-Services/index.html. The CMS Nursing Home Compare Provider Information files were accessed on Oct. 30, 2018, from https://data.medicare.gov/data/ archives/nursing-home-compare.

[72] As part of our data reliability checks, we matched the abuse deficiencies associated with the narrative descriptions in CMS's Automated Survey Processing Environment database with the abuse deficiencies in CMS's Certification and Survey Provider Enhanced Reports system. We found that we were unable to find matches for a relatively small number of records. CMS attributed these mismatches to differences in the source data used for the datasets. Specifically, state survey agencies enter data into the Automated Survey Processing Environment database, and that information is then uploaded by the states to CMS. These data from the states are then fed into CMS's Certification and Survey Provider Enhanced Reports system. In addition, officials said that there are some situations in which an abuse deficiency would not result in a narrative description written by surveyors. Correspondingly, there are some situations where a narrative description would be written by surveyors but not be uploaded by the state survey agency to CMS.

sample of 400 narratives, and each narrative was reviewed by two separate reviewers who independently analyzed the text of each narrative to determine the abuse and perpetrator type according to the definitions that CMS implemented on November 28, 2017, in its State Operations Manual.[73] Any disagreements between the two reviewers were resolved by a third independent reviewer. (See Table 7.) For those narratives where the abuse type could not reasonably be categorized under an existing CMS definition, reviewers had the option to mark narratives as "other." Furthermore, we analyzed the scope and severity for each narrative within our sample.

CMS's abuse deficiency code also included involuntary seclusion in the time period we examined and is defined in its November 22, 2017, guidance as "separation of a resident from other residents or from her/his room or confinement to her/his room (with or without roommates) against the resident's will, or the will of the resident representative."[74] Our analysis of the narrative descriptions found that 3 percent of the abuse deficiency narratives in our sample were attributable to involuntary seclusion. We were unable to categorize the abuse and perpetrator type for about 11 percent of the deficiency narratives in our sample, because we determined the narrative description did not meet CMS's abuse definition.

---

[73] We chose to use the definitions in CMS's current guidance for our narrative analysis despite the fact that they are more specific than the definitions in the CMS guidance that were in place at the time the narratives were written, because the specificity of the definitions in the current guidance allowed for us to perform a more consistent and reliable content analysis. For example, the older CMS guidance defines sexual abuse as "includes, but is not limited to, sexual harassment, sexual coercion, or sexual assault," while the newer guidance that we used for our analysis defines it as "includes, but is not limited to: unwanted intimate touching of any kind especially of breasts or perineal area, all types of sexual assault or battery, such as rape, sodomy, and coerced nudity, forced observation of masturbation and/or pornography, and taking sexually explicit photographs and/or audio/video recordings and maintaining and/or distributing them." Using CMS's updated definition of these terms provides internal validity by assuring reviewers followed CMS's contiguous approach to the proper use of these terms. CMS, *State Operations Manual, Appendix PP – Guidance to Surveyors for Long Term Care Facilities*. (November 22, 2017).

[74] CMS. *State Operations Manual, Appendix PP—Guidance to Surveyors for Long Term Care Facilities*. (November 22, 2017).

Table 7. Centers for Medicare & Medicaid Services' (CMS) Abuse and Perpetrator Type Definitions

Abuse type	CMS definition
Physical	Physical abuse includes, but is not limited to, hitting, slapping, punching, biting, and kicking. This definition includes corporal punishment, which includes, but is not limited to, pinching, spanking, slapping of hands, flicking, or hitting with an object.
Mental/verbal	Mental abuse is the use of verbal or nonverbal conduct which causes or has the potential to cause the resident to experience humiliation, intimidation, fear, shame, agitation, or degradation. Verbal abuse may be considered to be a type of mental abuse. Verbal abuse includes the use of oral, written, or gestured communication, or sounds, to residents within hearing distance, regardless of age, ability to comprehend, or disability.
Sexual	Sexual abuse is non-consensual sexual contact of any type with a resident and includes, but is not limited to: • Unwanted intimate touching of any kind especially of breasts or perineal area; • All types of sexual assault or battery, such as rape, sodomy, and coerced nudity; • Forced observation of masturbation and/or pornography; and • Taking sexually explicit photographs and/or audio/video recordings of a resident(s) and maintaining and/or distributing them (e.g., posting on social media). This would include, but is not limited to, nudity, fondling, and/or intercourse involving a resident.
Staff	Staff perpetrators are perpetrators who are staff, at any level, of the nursing facility.
Resident	Resident perpetrators are perpetrators who are also residents at the facility.
Other	Other perpetrators are perpetrators who do not fall into the previous two categories, and can include but are not limited to family members of residents, visitors, or strangers.

Source: CMS, State Operations Manual, Appendix PP—Guidance to Surveyors for Long Term Care Facilities. (November 22, 2017). | GAO-19-433.

We assessed the reliability of each of the datasets by checking for missing values and obvious errors and discussed them with CMS officials who were knowledgeable about the data. In the course of this assessment, we found some data limitations. Specifically, CMS officials told us that some state survey agencies may not have entered all facility- reported incidents into the Automated Survey Processing Environment Complaint/Incident Tracking System, while other state survey agencies did.[75] We also found underreporting, as noted in our 2019 report, where the Oregon state survey agency was not entering all abuse-related complaints

[75] CMS guidance requires state survey agencies to enter facility-reported incidents into the CMS database that require a federal, on-site survey.

or facility-reported incidents into this same database—a problem that could exist in other states.[76] In addition, CMS officials told us that it is possible there are additional incidents that may not have been represented in the abuse deficiency data during the period of our review. Specifically, CMS officials noted that some incidents resulting from resident altercations—particularly those that do not show a willful intent to harm—may not be cited as an abuse deficiency by some state survey agencies. We therefore consider the number of abuse deficiencies that resulted from complaints or facility-reported incidents to be a conservative estimate. After reviewing the possible limitations of these data, we determined the data were sufficiently reliable for the purposes of this reporting objective.

APPENDIX II: TRENDS IN ABUSE- RELATED DEFICIENCIES

This appendix describes trends in abuse-related deficiencies over the 5-year period from 2013 through 2017. We reviewed Centers for Medicare & Medicaid Services (CMS) guidance that was in effect during this period of review to determine which federal standards and deficiency codes were relevant to resident abuse.[77] For the report, we focused our analysis on the deficiency code cited when state surveyors substantiate incidents of abuse, but there are also deficiencies that surveyors can cite for abuse-related

---

[76] See GAO-19-313R. Further, our 2011 report noted CMS's concerns regarding the underreporting of complaints from state survey agencies. See GAO, *Nursing Homes: More Reliable Data and Consistent Guidance Would Improve CMS Oversight of State Complaint Investigations*, GAO-11-280, (Washington, D.C.: Apr. 7, 2011).

[77] Specifically, we reviewed Appendix PP of the State Operations Manual because it is the section that provides guidance to state surveyors about determining compliance with federal quality standards and their associated deficiency codes. There were multiple updates to Appendix PP of the State Operations Manual during the period of our review (January 1, 2013 through November 27, 2017). Specifically, there were eight updates to the appendix during the 5-year period, but none of these changed the abuse deficiency citation codes used by state surveyors. Therefore, we used the March 8, 2017, version of the Appendix PP—the most recent version during our period of review—when determining which deficiency codes to analyze for this report. CMS restructured its deficiency code system beginning on November 28, 2017, and, due to these coding changes, we did not analyze CMS data recorded by surveyors after the implementation of that change. CMS, *State Operations Manual, Appendix PP—Guidance to Surveyors for Long Term Care Facilities*. (March 8, 2017).

issues, such as a failure by the nursing home to train staff on issues related to abuse, either in conjunction with an abuse deficiency or without an abuse deficiency. Since these abuse-related deficiencies do not necessarily represent incidents of abuse, but do represent situations where a nursing home's inadequate policies could leave residents vulnerable to abuse, we also conducted a limited analysis on the trends of these deficiencies. Specifically, we analyzed CMS data to identify the number of abuse-related deficiencies cited in each year in all 50 states and Washington, D.C., and determined how many were cited at each level of severity—no actual harm with a potential for minimal harm, no actual harm with a potential for more than minimal harm, actual harm, and immediate jeopardy.[78] We also tracked the source of these abuse-related deficiencies—that is, whether the deficiency originated from a standard survey, complaint investigation, or a facility-reported incident investigation.[79] Finally, we compared the results for abuse-related deficiencies with the results for all types of deficiencies cited by surveyors in each year.

From 2013 to 2017, we found that abuse-related deficiencies became slightly more common with a resulting increase in severity. Specifically, abuse-related deficiencies increased by about 9.9 percent over the 5-year period, from 4,899 deficiencies cited in 2013 to 5,383 deficiencies cited in

---

[78] We analyzed data provided by CMS from its Certification and Survey Provider Enhanced Reports system. To avoid over-counting deficiencies, deficiencies that were for the same violation on the same day for the same facility were counted as a single deficiency. For example, there are instances where a complaint is filed and the complaint investigation window coincides with a scheduled standard survey. CMS data records the deficiency as two separate records—as the result of a standard survey and as the result of a complaint investigation. Following CMS procedure, we counted this deficiency only once; however, we flagged that the deficiency resulted from a complaint and a standard survey. Consequently, the sum of the source of the deficiencies (complaint investigation, facility-reported incident investigation, and standard survey) will be greater than the number of deficiencies.

[79] We matched the deficiencies with data provided by CMS from its Automated Survey Processing Environment Complaint/Incident Tracking System using provider number, survey date, and deficiency code. We found that some deficiencies were the result of a combination of complaint investigations, facility-reported incident investigations, standard surveys, or all three. We counted those deficiencies as originating from each relevant category.

2017, but peaked in 2016 with 5,687 deficiencies.[80] This increasing trend for abuse-related deficiencies is in contrast to the slight decrease in all deficiencies cited over the same period, but not nearly as high as the 103.5 percent increase in abuse deficiencies. In addition, the proportion of abuse-related deficiencies cited at the highest levels of severity— deficiencies causing actual harm to residents or putting residents in immediate jeopardy—fluctuated throughout the 5-year period. Specifically, about 6.1 percent of the 4,899 abuse-related deficiencies in 2013, about 5.6 percent of the 5,278 abuse-related deficiencies in 2015, and about 7.8 percent of the 5,383 abuse-related deficiencies in 2017 caused actual harm or immediate jeopardy.[81] (See Figure 7.)

We also found that over half of the abuse-related deficiencies each year were cited by surveyors as a result of standard surveys, and the rest were cited by surveyors as a result of either complaint or facility-reported incident investigations.[82] This falls between what we found for abuse deficiencies—the majority were a result of either complaint or facility-reported incident investigations—and all types of deficiencies—the vast majority were a result of standard surveys. Over the 5 years, similar to abuse deficiencies and all types of deficiencies, the percentage of abuse-related deficiencies that resulted from standard surveys decreased while the percentage that resulted from both complaint and facility-reported incident investigations increased. Specifically, over the 5-year period, the percentage of abuse-related deficiencies resulting from standard surveys decreased by about 8.8 percentage points, complaint investigations

[80] Similarly, the number of nursing homes that had abuse-related deficiencies cited also increased over the 5-year period from 3,318 (about 22.4 percent of all surveyed nursing homes) in 2013 to 3,563 (about 24.5 percent of all surveyed nursing homes) in 2017, but peaked in 2016 with 3,760 nursing homes (about 25.1 percent of all surveyed nursing homes) cited with abuse-related deficiencies. A nursing home can have more than one abuse-related deficiency cited within a single year.

[81] Abuse-related deficiencies were categorized by scope fairly consistently each year, with about two-thirds of abuse-related deficiencies categorized as isolated, about one-quarter categorized as a pattern, and less than 9 percent categorized as widespread.

[82] For 4,275 of the 26,466 total abuse-related deficiencies cited from 2013 through 2017, we were unable to determine from CMS's data whether the deficiency was identified during a standard survey, complaint investigation, facility-reported incident investigation, or a combination. We excluded these deficiencies from our percentages.

increased by about 3.6 percentage points, and facility-reported incident investigations increased by about 5.3 percentage points. (See Figure 8.)

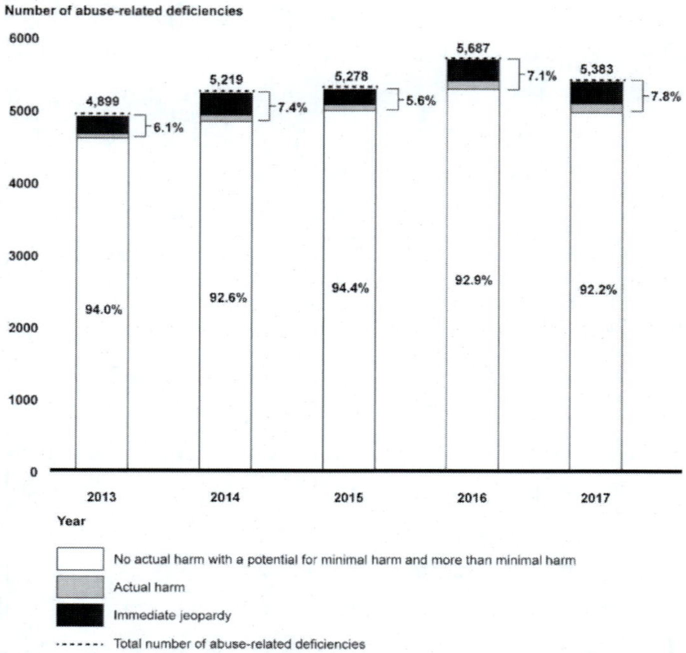

Source: GAO analysis of Centers for Medicare & Medicaid Services' (CMS) data. | GAO-19-433

Notes: CMS categorizes deficiencies into one of four severity categories based on whether the deficiency constitutes: (1) no actual harm with a potential for minimal harm; (2) no actual harm with a potential for more than minimal harm, but not immediate jeopardy; (3) actual harm that is not immediate jeopardy; or (4) immediate jeopardy to resident health or safety. We combined the first two categories in this figure.

CMS restructured its deficiency code system beginning on November 28, 2017, and, due to these coding changes, we did not analyze CMS data cited by surveyors after the implementation of that change.

Percentages may not add to 100 due to rounding.

Figure 7. Abuse-Related Deficiencies Cited, by Severity, 2013 through 2017.

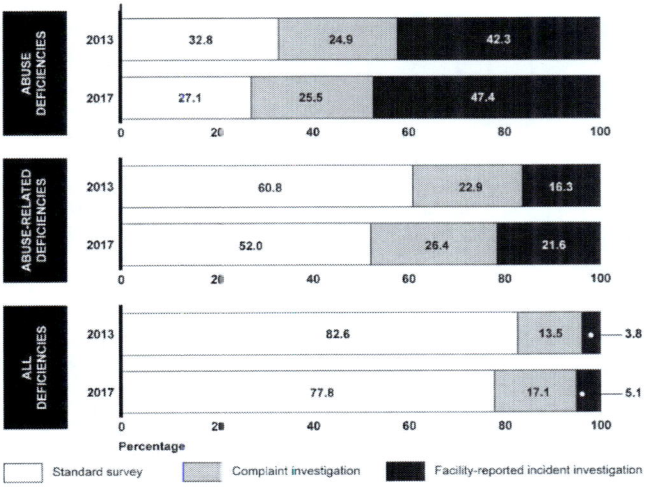

Source: GAO analysis of Centers for Medicare & Medicaid Services' (CMS) data. | GAO-19-433

Notes: For 375 out of 2,892 abuse deficiencies, 4,275 of the 26,466 abuse-related deficiencies, and 55,190 out of 538,559 total deficiencies cited over the time period, we were unable to determine from CMS's data whether the deficiency was identified during a standard survey, complaint investigation, facility-reported incident investigation, or a combination. We excluded these deficiencies from our percentages in the figure.

CMS restructured its deficiency code system beginning on November 28, 2017, and, due to these coding changes, we did not analyze CMS data cited by surveyors after the implementation of that change.

Percentages may not add to 100 due to rounding.

Figure 8. Source of Abuse Deficiencies, Abuse-Related Deficiencies, and All Types of Deficiencies, 2013 and 2017.

Appendix III: State Information on Abuse Deficiencies

Tables 8 and 9 provide state-level data on abuse deficiencies and the nursing homes that had abuse deficiencies cited in consecutive years.

Table 8. Abuse Deficiencies Cited, by State, 2013 and 2017

State	2013			2017[a]		
	Number of surveyed nursing homes	Number (percentage) of surveyed nursing homes with an abuse deficiency cited	Number (percentage) of cited deficiencies that were for abuse	Number of surveyed nursing homes	Number (percentage) of surveyed nursing homes with an abuse deficiency cited	Number (percentage) of cited deficiencies that were for abuse
AK	18	1 (5.6)	1 (0.5)	16	0 (0)	0 (0)
AL	220	1 (0.5)	1 (0.1)	201	0 (0)	0 (0)
AR	230	3 (1.3)	4 (0.3)	217	8 (3.7)	8 (0.6)
AZ	134	5 (3.7)	5 (0.5)	131	7 (5.3)	7 (1.5)
CA	1,164	73 (6.3)	85 (0.7)	1,174	75 (6.4)	82 (0.6)
CO	212	3 (1.4)	3 (0.2)	187	3 (1.6)	3 (0.2)
CT	227	31 (13.7)	33 (1.7)	213	32 (15.0)	34 (2.3)
DC	19	2 (10.5)	4 (1.4)	18	2 (11.1)	2 (1.1)
DE	43	2 (4.7)	2 (0.3)	40	1 (2.5)	1 (0.3)
FL	644	4 (0.6)	4 (0.1)	646	18 (2.8)	18 (0.5)
GA	268	0 (0)	0 (0)	325	5 (1.5)	5 (0.5)
HI	26	0 (0)	0 (0)	37	1 (2.7)	1 (0.3)
IA	415	1 (0.2)	1 (<0.1)	400	30 (7.5)	32 (1.9)
ID	72	0 (0)	0 (0)	61	1 (1.6)	2 (0.4)
IL	753	29 (3.9)	30 (0.6)	728	106 (14.6)	114 (1.7)
IN	501	25 (5.0)	26 (0.7)	535	53 (9.9)	55 (1.4)
KS	312	2 (0.6)	2 (<0.1)	269	27 (10.0)	28 (1.5)
KY	281	4 (1.4)	4 (0.3)	264	5 (1.9)	5 (0.4)
LA	279	4 (1.4)	4 (0.2)	267	5 (1.9)	5 (0.5)
MA	407	1 (0.3)	1 (<0.1)	380	15 (4.0)	16 (0.8)
MD	229	6 (2.6)	6 (0.2)	219	22 (10.0)	24 (1.0)
ME	101	0 (0)	0 (0)	100	1 (1.0)	1 (0.3)
MI	421	58 (13.8)	68 (1.7)	430	80 (18.6)	91 (1.8)
MN	350	1 (0.3)	1 (<0.1)	333	6 (1.8)	6 (0.3)
MO	491	1 (0.2)	1 (<0.1)	480	1 (0.2)	1 (<0.1)
MS	202	6 (3.0)	8 (0.6)	191	2 (1.1)	2 (0.3)
MT	77	2 (2.6)	2 (0.3)	61	2 (3.3)	2 (0.4)
NC	387	0 (0)	0 (0)	407	11 (2.7)	11 (0.5)
ND	78	0 (0)	0 (0)	69	0 (0)	0 (0)
NE	201	4 (2.0)	4 (0.3)	193	18 (9.3)	19 (1.5)
NH	73	1 (1.4)	1 (0.4)	69	0 (0)	0 (0)
NJ	351	4 (1.1)	4 (0.3)	334	0 (0)	0 (0)
NM	65	0 (0)	0 (0)	75	10 (13.3)	10 (1.2)
NV	50	1 (2.0)	1 (0.2)	59	1 (1.7)	1 (0.2)
NY	606	11 (1.8)	11 (0.3)	533	5 (0.9)	5 (0.2)
OH	862	56 (6.5)	58 (1.3)	901	79 (8.8)	85 (1.6)
OK	316	3 (1.0)	3 (<0.1)	283	11 (3.9)	11 (0.5)
OR	120	1 (0.8)	1 (0.2)b	129	2 (1.6)	2 (0.2)b
PA	690	2 (0.3)	2 (<0.1)	680	19 (2.8)	19 (0.3)
RI	78	0 (0)	0 (0)	79	0 (0)	0 (0)
SC	174	1 (0.6)	1 (0.1)	168	11 (6.6)	12 (1.0)
SD	100	2 (2.0)	2 (0.3)	96	0 (0)	0 (0)
TN	262	1 (0.4)	2 (0.1)	296	18 (6.1)	18 (1.3)

State	2013			2017[a]		
	Number of surveyed nursing homes	Number (percentage) of surveyed nursing homes with an abuse deficiency cited	Number (percentage) of cited deficiencies that were for abuse	Number of surveyed nursing homes	Number (percentage) of surveyed nursing homes with an abuse deficiency cited	Number (percentage) of cited deficiencies that were for abuse
TX	1,161	8 (0.7)	8 (<0.1)	1,166	89 (7.6)	97 (1.2)
UT	92	0 (0)	0 (0)	80	2 (2.5)	2 (0.3)
VA	279	10 (3.6)	10 (0.4)	263	6 (2.3)	6 (0.3)
VT	36	11 (30.6)	13 (4.2)	36	2 (5.6)	3 (1.4)
WA	216	2 (0.9)	2 (0.1)	219	16 (7.3)	16 (0.6)
WI	372	9 (2.4)	9 (0.3)	351	7 (2.0)	7 (0.3)
WV	105	2 (1.9)	2 (0.2)	104	5 (4.8)	5 (0.5)
WY	36	0 (0)	0 (0)	37	1 (2.7)	1 (0.3)
Total	**14,806**	**394 (2.7)**	**430 (0.4)**	**14,550**	**821 (5.6)**	**875 (0.8)**

Source: GAO analysis of Centers for Medicare & Medicaid Services' (CMS) data. | GAO-19-433.

Notes:

[a] CMS restructured its deficiency code system beginning on November 28, 2017, and, due to these coding changes, we did not analyze CMS data cited by surveyors after the implementation of that change.

[b] Our analysis of CMS data for Oregon does not include abuse deficiencies that may have resulted from investigations of complaints and facility-reported incidents. Specifically, we previously reported that Oregon was not following federal requirements that the state survey agency investigate all complaints and facility-reported incidents. Instead, for at least 15 years, Oregon's Adult Protective Services investigated complaints and facility-reported incidents of abuse in nursing homes and the results of those investigations were not shared with CMS. See GAO-19-313R.

Table 9. Nursing Homes with Abuse Deficiencies Cited in Consecutive Years, by State, 2013 through 2017

State	Total surveyed nursing homes, 2013 - 2017	Nursing homes with abuse deficiencies cited in only 1 year	Nursing homes with abuse deficiencies cited in multiple nonconsecutive years	Nursing homes with abuse deficiencies cited in two consecutive years	Nursing homes with abuse deficiencies cited in 3 or more consecutive years
AK	18	1	—	1	—
AL	232	5	—	—	—
AR	243	17	—	1	—
AZ	149	37	1	5	1
CA	1,258	225	33	29	9
CO	228	11	1	1	—
CT	231	74	11	15	1
DC	20	5	1	1	—
DE	47	6	1	—	—
FL	699	32	—	—	—
GA	365	14	—	1	—
HI	48	1	—	—	—
IA	460	78	3	14	—
ID	79	2	—	—	—

Table 9. (Continued)

State	Total surveyed nursing homes, 2013 - 2017	Nursing homes with abuse deficiencies cited in only 1 year	Nursing homes with abuse deficiencies cited in multiple nonconsecutive years	Nursing homes with abuse deficiencies cited in two consecutive years	Nursing homes with abuse deficiencies cited in 3 or more consecutive years
IL	791	141	21	15	1
IN	567	123	13	10	2
KS	369	68	2	7	—
KY	293	33	—	—	—
LA	280	17	1	—	—
MA	427	32	—	—	—
MD	234	38	3	4	—
ME	108	5	—	—	—
MI	456	101	33	29	7
MN	392	14	—	—	—
MO	531	11	—	—	—
MS	214	18	—	—	—
MT	84	13	1	1	—
NC	433	29	—	—	—
ND	82	5	—	—	—
NE	233	30	6	4	—
NH	77	4	—	—	—
NJ	374	18	1	—	—
NM	80	16	2	2	—
NV	60	2	—	1	—
NY	637	27	—	1	—
OH	995	184	25	23	4
OK	333	27	2	—	—
OR	144	5	—	—	—
PA	716	30	1	3	—
RI	84	1	—	—	—
SC	192	20	2	1	—
SD	113	9	1	1	—
TN	337	29	1	1	—
TX	1,303	153	4	4	—
UT	105	7	—	—	—
VA	298	26	—	2	—
VT	38	7	4	4	—
WA	230	22	3	1	—
WI	409	33	—	2	—
WV	129	19	1	1	—
WY	41	1	—	—	—
Total	**16,266**	**1,826**	**178**	**185**	**25**

Legend: "—" = none.

Source: GAO analysis of Centers for Medicare & Medicaid Services' (CMS) data. | GAO-19-433.

Note: CMS restructured its deficiency code system beginning on November 28, 2017, and, due to these coding changes, we did not analyze CMS data cited by surveyors after the implementation of that change.

APPENDIX IV: COMMENTS FROM THE DEPARTMENT OF HEALTH AND HUMAN SERVICES

DEPARTMENT OF HEALTH & HUMAN SERVICES

OFFICE OF THE SECRETARY

Assistant Secretary for Legislation
Washington, DC 20201

MAY 22 2019

John Dicken
Director, Health Care
U.S. Government Accountability Office
441 G Street NW
Washington, DC 20548

Dear Mr. Dicken:

Attached are comments on the U.S. Government Accountability Office's (GAO) report entitled, "*Nursing Homes: Improved Oversight Needed to Better Protect Residents from Abuse*" (GAO-19-433).

The Department appreciates the opportunity to review this report prior to publication.

Sincerely,

Matthew D. Bassett
Assistant Secretary for Legislation

GENERAL COMMENTS FROM THE DEPARTMENT OF HEALTH & HUMAN SERVICES ON THE GOVERNMENT ACCOUNTABILITY OFFICE'S DRAFT REPORT ENTITLED - NURSING HOMES: IMPROVED OVERSIGHT NEEDED TO BETTER PROTECT RESIDENTS FROM ABUSE (GAO-19-433)

The U.S. Department of Health & Human Services (HHS) appreciates the opportunity to review and comment on the Government Accountability Office (GAO) draft report on the federal oversight of nursing homes. Resident safety in nursing homes and in all facilities that participate in the Medicare and Medicaid programs is a top priority for HHS.

Every nursing home resident deserves to retain their basic human dignity and to be treated with respect at all times. Abuse and neglect are never acceptable. HHS is undertaking a comprehensive review of the regulations, guidelines, internal structure, and processes related to safety and quality in nursing homes. HHS has demonstrated a commitment to this path by developing a five-part plan to ensure the care provided in nursing homes is of the highest possible quality. The five-part plan will strengthen oversight, enhance enforcement, increase transparency, improve quality, and put patients over paperwork.

HHS works in partnership with state survey agencies to oversee nursing homes, since these agencies are generally also responsible for state licensure. The state survey agencies visit and conduct survey inspections at every Medicare and Medicaid participating nursing home in the nation at least annually to ensure they are meeting HHS' health and safety requirements as well as state licensure requirements. State survey agencies can also conduct complaint surveys at any time, and anyone can file a complaint, including residents, family members, nursing home staff, and anyone else who has reason to suspect abuse or neglect is taking place. HHS's Nursing Home Compare website includes links and other helpful information to help patients and families determine when and how to file a complaint. Nursing homes are required to post similar information on how to file complaints and grievances in their facilities and with independent state entities. HHS will be updating Nursing Home Compare to make it easier for consumers to identify specific instances of non-compliance related to abuse.

Residents deserve consistent nursing home quality, regardless of location, so HHS is revising its oversight of state survey agency performance. HHS is examining the way surveyors identify issues such as abuse, facility staffing levels, and dementia care, and is clarifying expectations regarding when abuse must be reported to the state and law enforcement. This means setting clear timelines for state survey agencies to review allegations of abuse and neglect.

In addition, HHS conducts validation surveys to determine whether state survey agencies are identifying deficiencies correctly, investigating compliance effectively, and meeting all other obligations. The Centers for Medicare & Medicaid Services (CMS) Regional Offices conduct formal assessments annually of each state survey agency's performance relative to measures included in the State Performance Standards System (SPSS). The SPSS provides a framework to organize and measure important aspects of state survey activities and is comprised of three domains: frequency, survey quality, and enforcement. These three areas also support HHS's efforts to standardize and promote consistency among state survey agencies.

HHS recently revised the process for validation surveys conducted of state survey agencies to add areas of concern that federal surveyors will examine to determine whether state surveyors are investigating for compliance effectively. In fiscal year 2018, HHS worked with states on three areas of concern: abuse and neglect, admission/transfer/discharge, and dementia care. In 2019, each Regional Office will again focus on identifying concerns related to abuse and neglect. They will also focus on facility staffing and other areas of improvement that are unique to the states in its region. HHS also recently launched an initiative to evaluate the entire SPSS program to identify ways to improve state performance. This is an ongoing, large-scale effort aimed at improving the efficiency and effectiveness of measuring and improving state performance.

HHS remains diligent in our duties to monitor nursing homes participating in Medicare and Medicaid across the country, as well as the state agencies that survey them. HHS appreciates the ongoing work of the GAO in this area and will continue to work with them as we make improvements to our oversight efforts.

GAO's recommendations and HHS' responses are below.

Recommendation 1
Require that abuse and perpetrator type be submitted by state survey agencies in CMS's databases for deficiency, complaint, and facility-reported incident data and that CMS systematically assess trends in these data.

HHS Response
HHS concurs with this recommendation. HHS requires state survey agencies to investigate and track complaints of abuse and neglect at nursing homes and will look into options for requiring state agencies to record alleged abuse type and alleged perpetrator type, when available, so that HHS may assess trends in these data.

Recommendation 2
Develop and disseminate guidance—including a standardized form—to all survey agencies on the information nursing homes and covered individuals should include on facility-reported incidents.

HHS Response
HHS concurs with this recommendation. HHS has training materials for state agency and nursing home staff on identifying and reporting potential abuse and neglect of beneficiaries and already has plans to issue new guidance specific to the reporting and tracking of facility-reported incidents of potential abuse and neglect. HHS will develop a list of standardized data elements that must be included when reporting facility-reported incidents to state survey agencies. Since reporting forms

vary depending on state laws and requirements, rather than creating a standardized form, HHS will provide guidance that any reporting form should include all of the standardized elements required by HHS.

Recommendation 3
Require state survey agencies to immediately refer complaints and surveys to law enforcement (and, when applicable, to MFCUs) if they have a reasonable suspicion that a crime against a resident has occurred when the complaint is received.

HHS Response
HHS concurs with this recommendation. Currently, state survey agencies are required to investigate and track complaints of abuse and neglect and report substantiated findings to local law enforcement and MFCUs when appropriate (CMS State Operations Manual, § 5330). In the case of alleged violations involving abuse, neglect, exploitation or mistreatment in a nursing facility, HHS requires the facility to report to the state survey agency and adult protective services where state law provides for jurisdiction in long term care facilities in accordance with state law through established procedures (42 CFR 483.12). In cases where the state survey agency cannot verify that the facility already reported to law enforcement, HHS will require state survey agencies to immediately refer complaints to law enforcement if a reasonable suspicion of a crime against a resident has occurred and share any subsequent relevant survey information.

Recommendation 4
Conduct oversight of state survey agencies to ensure referrals of complaints, surveys, and substantiated incidents with reasonable suspicion of a crime are referred to law enforcement (and, when applicable, MFCUs) in a timely fashion.

HHS Response
HHS concurs with this recommendation. HHS requires state survey agencies to investigate and track complaints of abuse and neglect and report substantiated findings to local law enforcement (CMS State Operations Manual, § 5330); however, we will consider how to implement mechanisms for tracking law enforcement referrals.

Recommendation 5
Develop guidance for state survey agencies clarifying that allegations verified by evidence should be substantiated and reported to law enforcement and state registries in cases where citing a federal deficiency may not be appropriate.

HHS Response
HHS concurs with this recommendation. Nursing homes are required under 42 CFR 483.12 to report alleged violations of abuse, neglect, exploitation, or mistreatment of residents to the appropriate authorities; however, HHS will review our guidance to state agencies for opportunities to provide additional clarification around allegations where a federal deficiency may not be appropriate..

Recommendation 6
Provide guidance on what information should be contained in the referral of abuse allegations to law enforcement.

HHS Response
HHS concurs with this recommendation. HHS will provide guidance to state agencies and nursing homes on identifying and reporting potential abuse and neglect of residents and will develop a list of standardized elements that should be included when reporting an abuse allegation to law enforcement.

APPENDIX V: ACCESSIBLE DATA

Data Tables

Data Table for Figure 2: Severity of Cited Abuse Deficiencies, 2013 through 2017

Year	No actual harm with a potential for minimal harm and more than minimal harm		Actual harm		Immediate jeopardy		Combination of actual harm and immediate jeopardy		Total number of abuse deficiencies
	Number of abuse deficiencies	Percentage of abuse deficiencies	Number of abuse deficiencies	Percentage of abuse deficiencies	Number of abuse deficiencies	Percentage of abuse deficiencies	Number of abuse deficiencies	Percentage of abuse deficiencies	
2013	293	68.1	69	16.0	68	15.8	137	31.9	430
2014	269	60.9	102	23.1	71	16.1	173	39.1	442
2015	296	64.6	92	20.1	70	15.3	162	35.4	458
2016	390	56.8	186	27.1	111	16.2	297	43.2	687
2017	502	57.4	196	22.4	177	20.2	373	42.6	875

Data Table for Figure 3: Type of Survey or Investigation Used to Identify Abuse Deficiencies and All Types of Deficiencies, 2013 through 2017

Deficiency	Year	Standard survey	Complaint investigation	Facility-reported incident investigation
Abuse deficiencies	2013	32.8	24.9	42.3
	2014	33.3	27.1	39.6
	2015	33.3	24.1	42.7
	2016	29.0	22.6	48.4
	2017	27.1	25.5	47.4
All deficiencies	2013	82.6	13.5	3.8
	2014	80.6	15.0	4.4
	2015	80.9	15.1	4.0
	2016	78.4	17.1	4.6
	2017	77.8	17.1	5.1

Data Table for Figure 4: Types of Implemented Enforcement Actions for Abuse Deficiencies, 2013 through 2017

Year	Civil money penalty	Denial of payment for new Medicare or Medicaid admissions	Mandatory termination from the Medicare and Medicaid programs	Other remedies
2013	16 (69.6%)	8 (34.8%)	0	0
2014	20 (83.3%)	5 (20.8%)	1 (4.2%)	0
2015	19 (76.0%)	5 (20.0%)	0	1 (4.0%)
2016	39 (79.6%)	10 (20.4%)	0	2 (4.1%)
2017	54 (83.1%)	9 (13.8%)	0	5 (7.7%)

Data Table for Figure 7: Abuse-Related Deficiencies Cited, by Severity, 2013 through 2017

Year	No actual harm with a potential for minimal harm and more than minimal harm		Actual harm	Immediate jeopardy	Combination of actual harm and immediate jeopardy		Total number of abuse-related deficiencies
	Number of abuse-related deficiencies	Percentage of abuse-related deficiencies	Number of abuse-related deficiencies	Number of abuse-related deficiencies	Number of abuse-related deficiencies	Percentage of abuse-related deficiencies	
2013	4,603	94.0	56	241	297	6.1	4,899
2014	4,834	92.6	86	300	386	7.4	5.219
2015	4,981	94.4	87	210	297	5.6	5,278
2016	5,286	92.9	112	289	401	7.1	5,687
2017	4,964	92.2	121	298	419	7.8	5,383

Data Table for Figure 8: Source of Abuse Deficiencies, Abuse-Related Deficiencies, and All Types of Deficiencies, 2013 and 2017

Deficiency	Year	Standard survey	Complaint investigation	Facility-reported incident investigation
Abuse deficiencies	2013	32.8	24.9	42.3
	2017	27.1	25.5	47.4
Abuse-related deficiencies	2013	60.8	22.9	16.3
	2017	52.0	26.4	21.6
All deficiencies	2013	82.6	13.5	3.8
	2017	77.8	17.1	5.1

In: Nursing Homes and Elder Abuse
Editor: Joshua Newland
ISBN: 978-1-53617-974-3
© 2020 Nova Science Publishers, Inc.

Chapter 3

NURSING HOMES: BETTER OVERSIGHT NEEDED TO PROTECT RESIDENTS FROM ABUSE*

John E. Dicken

WHY GAO DID THIS STUDY

Nationwide, about 1.4 million elderly or disabled individuals receive care in more than 15,500 nursing homes. CMS, an agency within the Department of Health and Human Services (HHS), defines standards nursing homes must meet to participate in the Medicare and Medicaid programs.

Nursing home residents often have physical or cognitive limitations that can leave them particularly vulnerable to abuse. Abuse of nursing home residents can occur in many forms—including physical, mental, verbal, and sexual— and can be committed by staff, residents, or others in the nursing home. Any incident of abuse is a serious occurrence and can

* This is an edited, reformatted and augmented version of the United States Government Accountability Office Statement for the Record to the Committee on Ways and Means, House of Representatives, Publication No. GAO-20-259T, dated November 14, 2019.

result in potentially devastating consequences for residents, including lasting mental anguish, serious injury, or death.

This statement summarizes GAO's June 2019 report, GAO-19-433. Specifically, it describes: (1) the trends and types of abuse in recent years, and (2) CMS's oversight intended to ensure residents are free from abuse. It also includes a brief summary of findings and recommendations from this June 2019 report and prior GAO reports that examined the health and welfare of the elderly in multiple settings, and the status, as of November 2019, of HHS's efforts to implement the recommendations GAO made.

WHAT GAO FOUND

The Centers for Medicare & Medicaid Services (CMS) is responsible for ensuring nursing homes meet federal quality standards, including that residents are free from abuse. CMS enters into agreements with state survey agencies to conduct surveys of the state's homes and to investigate complaints and incidents.

GAO's June 2019 report found that, while abuse deficiencies cited in nursing homes were relatively rare from 2013 through 2017, they more than doubled during that time, increasing from 430 in 2013 to 875 in 2017, with the largest increase in severe cases. In light of the increased number and severity of abuse deficiencies, it is imperative that CMS have strong nursing home oversight in place to protect residents from abuse. However, GAO found oversight gaps that may limit the agency's ability to do so. Specifically, GAO found:

- *Information on abuse and perpetrator types is not readily available.* CMS's data do not allow for the type of abuse or perpetrator to be readily identified by the agency. Specifically, CMS does not require the state survey agencies to record abuse and perpetrator type and, when this information is recorded, it cannot be easily analyzed by CMS. GAO made a recommendation that CMS require state survey agencies to submit data on abuse and perpetrator type and HHS concurred. As of November 2019, HHS had not implemented the recommendation.

- *Facility-reported incidents lack key information.* Despite federal law requiring nursing homes to self-report allegations of abuse and covered individuals to report reasonable suspicions of crimes against residents, CMS has not provided guidance to nursing homes on what information they should include in facility-reported incidents, contributing to a lack of information for state survey agencies and delays in their investigations. GAO made a recommendation that CMS develop guidance on what abuse information nursing homes should self-report and HHS concurred. As of November 2019, HHS had not implemented the recommendation.
- *Gaps exist in the CMS process for state survey agency referrals to law enforcement.* GAO found gaps in CMS's process for referring incidents of abuse to law enforcement. These gaps may limit CMS's ability to ensure that nursing homes meet federal requirements for residents to be free from abuse. Specifically, GAO identified issues related to (1) referring abuse to law enforcement in a timely manner, (2) tracking abuse referrals, (3) defining what it means to substantiate an allegation of abuse—that is, the determination by the state survey agency that evidence supports the abuse allegation, and (4) sharing information with law enforcement. GAO made four recommendations to address these gaps and HHS concurred. As of November 2019, HHS had not implemented these recommendations.

Chairman Neal, Ranking Member Brady, and Members of the Committee:

I am pleased to submit this statement on GAO's work related to nursing home resident safety. Specifically, this statement discusses GAO's recent report on the abuse of nursing home residents and the Centers for

Medicare & Medicaid Services' (CMS) oversight.[1] Nationwide, about 1.4 million elderly or disabled individuals receive care in more than 15,500 nursing homes. These nursing home residents often have physical or cognitive limitations that can leave them particularly vulnerable to abuse. Abuse of nursing home residents can occur in many forms—including physical, mental, verbal, and sexual—and can be committed by staff, residents, or others in the nursing home. Any incident of abuse is a serious occurrence and can result in potentially devastating consequences for residents, including lasting mental anguish, serious injury, or death. News stories in recent years have noted disturbing examples of nursing home residents who have been sexually assaulted and physically abused. However, little is known about the full scope of nursing home abuse, as incidents of abuse may be underreported.

Federal law mandates that nursing homes receiving Medicare or Medicaid payments ensure that residents are free from abuse. To help ensure this, CMS, an agency within the Department of Health and Human Services (HHS), defines the quality standards that nursing homes must meet in order to participate in the Medicare and Medicaid programs.[2] To monitor compliance with these standards, CMS enters into agreements with agencies in each state government—known as state survey agencies—and oversees the work the state survey agencies do. This work includes conducting required, comprehensive, on-site standard surveys of every nursing home approximately once each year and investigating both complaints from the public and incidents self-reported by the nursing home (referred to as facility-reported incidents) regarding resident care or safety.[3]

---

[1] GAO, *Nursing Homes: Improved Oversight Needed to Better Protect Residents from Abuse*. GAO-19-433 (Washington, D.C.: June 13, 2019).

[2] CMS defines abuse in its guidance, the State Operations Manual (dated November 22, 2017), as "the willful infliction of injury, unreasonable confinement, intimidation, or punishment with resulting physical harm, pain or mental anguish. Abuse also includes the deprivation by an individual, including a caretaker, of goods or services that are necessary to attain or maintain physical, mental, and psychosocial well-being." This statement addresses physical abuse, mental and verbal abuse—which we refer to as "mental/verbal abuse"—and sexual abuse but does not address other forms of abuse, such as financial abuse or neglect.

[3] By law, every nursing home receiving Medicare or Medicaid payment must undergo a standard survey at least once every fifteen months, with a statewide average interval for surveys not to exceed 12 months. 42 U.S.C. §§ 1395i-3(g)(1)(A), (g)(2)(A)(iii), 1396r(g)(1)(A), (g)(2)(A)(iii). State survey agencies are also required to investigate complaints and facility-

If a surveyor determines that a nursing home violated a federal standard during a survey or investigation, then the home receives a deficiency citation, also known as a deficiency. In addition to state survey agencies, there are other state and local agencies that may be involved in investigating abuse in nursing homes, including Adult Protective Services, local law enforcement, and Medicaid Fraud Control Units (MFCU) in each state, which are tasked with investigating and prosecuting a variety of health care-related crimes.

We have previously reported on problems in nursing home quality, including challenges protecting residents from abuse and weaknesses in CMS's oversight. For example, in multiple reports dating back to 1998, we have identified weaknesses in federal and state activities designed to correct quality problems in nursing homes. Specifically, in a 2002 report, we found that CMS needed to do more to protect nursing home residents from abuse, and we made five recommendations to help CMS facilitate the reporting, investigation, and prevention of abuse in nursing homes.[4] More recently, in April 2019 we reported that CMS had failed to address gaps in federal oversight of nursing home abuse investigations in Oregon—an issue that we uncovered during the course of our broader work on nursing home resident abuse.[5] Further, reports by the HHS Office of the Inspector General (OIG) have also reviewed incidents of resident abuse and raised concerns about CMS's procedures.[6]

This statement highlights key findings and recommendations from our June 2019 report, which examined:

---

reported incidents filed with state survey agencies. 42 U.S.C. §§ 1395i-3(g)(1)(C), 1396r(g)(1)(C).

[4] CMS has implemented one of these recommendations—that CMS clarify the definition of abuse and otherwise ensure that states apply that definition consistently and appropriately. While CMS generally agreed with the other four recommendations, the agency did not implement the recommendations, and so we closed them as not implemented. See GAO, *Nursing Homes: More Can Be Done to Protect Residents from Abuse*, GAO-02-312, (Washington, D.C.: Mar. 1, 2002).

[5] GAO, Management Report: CMS Needs to Address Gaps in Federal Oversight of Nursing Home Abuse Investigations That Persisted in Oregon for at Least 15 Years, GAO- 19-313R, (Washington, D.C.: Apr. 15, 2019).

[6] For example, see Joanne M. Chiedi, Office of Inspector General, HHS, *Incidents of Potential Abuse and Neglect at Skilled Nursing Facilities Were Not Always Reported and Investigated*, A-01-16-00509 (Washington, D.C., June 7, 2019).

1. the trends and types of abuse occurring in nursing homes in recent years,
2. the risk factors for abuse and challenges facing stakeholder agencies involved in investigating abuse in nursing homes, and
3. CMS's oversight intended to ensure that nursing home residents are free from abuse.

In this statement, we include information on the status, as of November 2019, of HHS's efforts to implement the recommendations in our June 2019 report. In appendix I, we also include a summary of findings and recommendations from prior GAO reports that examined the health and welfare of the elderly in multiple settings, such as abuse in nursing homes, assisted living facilities, and in the community. A list of related GAO reports from our larger body of work examining federal oversight of the quality of care and the safety of older adults receiving care in these settings is included at the end of this statement.

To conduct the work for our June 2019 report, we reviewed federal laws and CMS guidance, analyzed CMS data, and interviewed stakeholders from selected states. First, we reviewed federal laws and CMS guidance to determine the federal standards and associated deficiency codes related to resident abuse. Second, we analyzed data provided by CMS to identify the number and severity of abuse deficiencies cited by surveyors in all 50 states and Washington, D.C., between 2013 and 2017.[7] Because abuse and perpetrator type are not readily identifiable in CMS's data, we identified this information by reviewing a randomly selected representative sample of 400 CMS abuse deficiency narratives written by state surveyors from 2016 through 2017 that describe the substantiated abuse.

---

[7] CMS restructured its deficiency code system beginning on November 28, 2017. Due to these coding changes, we did not analyze CMS data cited by surveyors after the implementation of that change.

Finally, we interviewed CMS officials and officials from a non-generalizable sample of survey agencies from five states—Delaware, Georgia, Ohio, Oregon, and Virginia. We also interviewed other stakeholders in these states, including officials from each state's long- term care ombudsmen, law enforcement, MFCUs, and, when appropriate, Adult Protective Services. We also visited nursing homes and spoke to administrators and clinical staff in each of these states. We assessed CMS's oversight activities in the context of the federal standards for internal control.[8] (Further details on our scope and methodology are included in our report). To determine the status of the recommendations we made in our June 2019 report, we obtained information from CMS officials in November 2019.

We conducted the work on which this statement is based in accordance with generally accepted government auditing standards. Those standards require that we plan and perform the audit to obtain sufficient, appropriate evidence to provide a reasonable basis for our findings and conclusions based on our audit objectives. We believe that the evidence obtained provides a reasonable basis for our findings and conclusions based on our audit objectives.

IMPROVED CMS OVERSIGHT IS NEEDED TO BETTER PROTECT RESIDENTS FROM ABUSE

In our June 2019 report, we found that, while abuse deficiencies cited in nursing homes were relatively rare from 2013 through 2017, they became more frequent during that time, with the largest increase in severe cases.

[8] GAO, *Standards for Internal Control in the Federal Government*. GAO-14-704G (Washington, D.C.: Sept. 10, 2014). Internal control is a process effected by an entity's oversight body, management, and other personnel that provides reasonable assurance that the objectives of an entity will be achieved.

Specifically, abuse deficiencies comprised less than 1 percent of the total deficiencies in each of the years we examined, which is likely conservative. Abuse in nursing homes is often underreported by residents, family, staff, and the state survey agency, according to CMS officials and stakeholders we interviewed. However, abuse deficiencies more than doubled—from 430 in 2013 to 875 in 2017—over the 5-year period.[9] (See appendix II.) In addition, abuse deficiencies cited in 2017 were more likely to be categorized at the highest levels of severity— deficiencies causing actual harm to residents or putting residents in immediate jeopardy—than they were in 2013. In light of the increased number and severity of abuse deficiencies, it is imperative that CMS have strong nursing home oversight in place to protect residents from abuse; however, we found oversight gaps that may limit the agency's ability to do so. Specifically, we found that CMS: (1) cannot readily access data on the type of abuse or type of perpetrator, (2) has not provided guidance on what information nursing homes should include in facility-reported incidents, and (3) has numerous gaps in its referral process that can result in delayed and missed referrals to law enforcement.

Information on Abuse and Perpetrator Types Is Not Readily Available

In our June 2019 report, we found that CMS's data do not allow for the type of abuse or perpetrator to be readily identified by the agency.

Specifically, CMS does not require the state survey agencies to record abuse and perpetrator type and, when this information is recorded, it cannot be easily analyzed by CMS.

[9] The trend for abuse deficiencies is in contrast to the trend across all types of deficiencies, which decreased about 1 percent between 2013 and 2017. Specifically, all deficiency types increased at a much slower rate than abuse deficiencies each year through 2016 and then decreased slightly through the period examined in 2017.

Therefore, we reviewed a representative sample of 400 CMS narrative descriptions—written by state surveyors—associated with abuse deficiencies cited in 2016 and 2017 to identify the most common types of abuse and perpetrators. From this review, we found that physical abuse (46 percent) and mental/verbal abuse (44 percent) occurred most often in nursing homes, followed by sexual abuse (18 percent).[10] Furthermore, staff, which includes those working in any part of the nursing home, were more often the perpetrators (58 percent) of abuse in deficiency narratives, followed by resident perpetrators (30 percent) and other types of perpetrators (2 percent).[11] (See appendix III for examples from our abuse deficiency narrative review.)

CMS officials told us they have not conducted a systematic review to gather information on abuse and perpetrator type. Further, based on professional experience, literature, and ad hoc analyses of deficiency narrative descriptions, CMS officials told us they believe the majority of abuse is committed by nursing home residents and that physical and sexual abuse were the most common types.[12] This understanding does not align with our findings on the most common types of abuse and perpetrators represented in CMS's data on deficiencies cited as abuse. Without the systematic collection and monitoring of specific abuse and perpetrator data, CMS lacks key information and, therefore, cannot take actions—such as tailoring prevention and investigation activities—to address the most prevalent types of abuse or perpetrators.[13] To address this, we

---

[10] Percentages may not add to 100 either because some narratives had multiple types of abuse, were missing or incomplete, or were not consistent with CMS's definition of abuse. Upper and lower confidence levels were: physical abuse (41 to 51 percent), mental/verbal abuse (40 to 49 percent), and sexual abuse (14 to 22 percent).

[11] Upper and lower confidence levels were: staff-on-resident abuse (54 to 63 percent), resident-on-resident abuse (26 to 35 percent), and abuse by others (1 to 3 percent). Other types of perpetrators can include family members of residents or other visitors.

[12] CMS officials noted that some incidents resulting from resident altercations—particularly those that do not show a willful intent to harm—may not have been cited as an abuse deficiency by some state survey agencies and may have been cited as other deficiencies not specified as abuse. This may have contributed to the difference between CMS's understanding of the prevalence of resident-to-resident abuse and what their abuse deficiency data show.

[13] The lack of a systematic review is also inconsistent with federal internal control standards directing management to use quality information to achieve program objectives. GAO-14-704G.

recommended that CMS require state survey agencies to report abuse and perpetrator type in CMS's databases for deficiency, complaint, and facility-reported incident data and that CMS systematically assess trends in these data. HHS concurred with our recommendation and stated that it plans to implement changes in response. As of November 2019, HHS had not implemented the recommendation.

Facility-Reported Incidents Lack Key Information

Despite federal law requiring nursing homes to self-report allegations of abuse and covered individuals to report reasonable suspicions of crimes against residents, in June 2019 we reported that CMS had not provided guidance to nursing homes on what information they should include in facility-reported incidents, contributing to a lack of information for state survey agencies and delays in their investigations.[14] Specifically, officials from each of the five state survey agencies told us that the documentation they receive from nursing homes for facility-reported incidents can lack key information that affects their ability to triage incidents and determine whether an investigation should occur and, if so, how soon. For example, officials from two state survey agencies we interviewed said they sometimes have to conduct significant follow-up with the nursing homes to obtain the information they need to prioritize the incident for investigation—follow-up that delays and potentially negatively affects investigations.[15] Incomplete incident reports from nursing homes are particularly problematic given that nearly half of abuse deficiencies cited between 2013 and 2017 were identified through facility-reported incidents, which is dramatically different than the approximately 5 percent of all types of deficiencies that were identified in this manner. Therefore, facility-reported incidents play a unique and significant role in identifying abuse

[14] 42 C.F.R. § 483.12(c)(1) (2018); 42 U.S.C. § 1320b-25(b). These covered individuals include nursing home owners, operators, and employees, among others.

[15] he lack of guidance from CMS on the information that state survey agencies should collect on facility-reported incidents is inconsistent with federal internal control standards directing management to use quality information to achieve program objectives. GAO-14- 704G.

deficiencies in nursing homes, making it critical that incident reports provided by nursing homes include the information necessary for state survey agencies to prioritize and investigate. To address this issue, we recommended that CMS develop and disseminate guidance— including a standardized form—to all state survey agencies on the information nursing homes and covered individuals should include on facility-reported incidents. HHS concurred with our recommendation and stated that it plans to implement changes in response. As of November 2019, HHS had not implemented the recommendation.

Gaps Exist in CMS Process for State Survey Agency Referrals to Law Enforcement and MFCUs

In June 2019, we identified gaps in CMS's process for referring incidents of abuse to law enforcement and, if appropriate, to MFCUs. These gaps may limit CMS's ability to ensure that nursing homes meet federal requirements for residents to be free from abuse. Specifically, we identified issues related to (1) referring abuse to law enforcement in a timely manner, (2) tracking abuse referrals, (3) defining what it means to substantiate an allegation of abuse—that is, the determination by the state survey agency that evidence supports the abuse allegation, and (4) sharing information with law enforcement. We made recommendations that CMS address each of these four gaps in the referral process, and HHS concurred with each recommendation and stated that it plans to implement changes in response. As of November 2019, HHS had not implemented these recommendations.

One of the gaps in CMS's process is related to referring abuse to law enforcement in a timely manner. For example, law enforcement investigations can be significantly delayed because CMS requires a state survey agency to make referrals to law enforcement only after abuse is substantiated—a process that can often take weeks or months. Officials from one law enforcement agency and two MFCUs we interviewed told us the delay in receiving referrals limits their ability to collect evidence and prosecute cases—for example, bedding associated with potential sexual abuse may have been washed, and a victim's wounds may have healed.[16] As such, we recommended that CMS require state survey agencies to immediately refer to law enforcement any reasonable suspicion of a crime against a resident. HHS concurred with our recommendation and stated that it plans to implement changes in response. As of November 2019, HHS had not implemented this recommendation.

In conclusion, while nursing home abuse is relatively rare, our June 2019 report shows that abuse deficiencies cited in nursing homes are becoming more frequent, with the largest increase in severe cases. It is imperative that CMS have more complete and readily available information on abuse to improve its oversight of nursing homes. It is also essential that CMS require state survey agencies to immediately report incidents to law enforcement if they have a reasonable suspicion that a crime against a resident has occurred in order to ensure a prompt investigation of these incidents.

Chairman Neal, Ranking Member Brady, and Members of the Committee, this concludes GAO's statement for the record.

Appendix I: Summary of GAO Reports on the Health and Welfare of the Elderly

We have issued a number of reports reviewing the health and welfare of the elderly in multiple settings. For example, since January 2015, we have issued reports on the incidence of abuse in nursing homes and what is known about the incidence of abuse in assisted living facilities. Reports often included key recommendations. (See table 1.)

[16] Such delays are inconsistent with standards for internal control, which state that management should communicate quality information externally so that external parties can help the entity achieve its objectives. GAO-14-704G.

Table 1. Examples of GAO reports reviewing the health and welfare of the elderly, January 2015-August 2019

Date	Title	Description
August 2019	*Elder Abuse: Federal Requirements for Oversight in Nursing Homes and Assisted Living Facilities Differ* (GAO-19-599)	GAO reviewed federal oversight of elder abuse reporting, investigation, and law enforcement notification in both nursing homes and assisted living facilities. GAO found that there are specific federal requirements for nursing homes and state survey agencies for reporting, investigating, and notifying law enforcement about elder abuse in nursing homes. In contrast, there are no similar federal requirements for assisted living facilities, which are licensed and regulated by states. Instead, the Centers for Medicare & Medicaid Services (CMS) requires state Medicaid agencies to develop policies to ensure the reporting and investigation of elder abuse in assisted living facilities. GAO did not make any recommendations. Setting: nursing homes and assisted living facilities
June 2019	*Nursing Homes: Improved Oversight Needed to Better Protect Residents from Abuse* (GAO-19-433)	GAO examined trends and types of abuse in nursing homes in recent years and CMS's oversight. GAO found that, while relatively rare, abuse deficiencies cited in nursing homes more than doubled from 2013 to 2017, and that gaps in CMS oversight may limit the agency's ability to protect residents from abuse. GAO made six recommendations including that CMS require state survey agencies to immediately notify law enforcement of any suspicion of a crime. The Department of Health and Human Services (HHS) agreed with the recommendations and, as of November 2019, HHS had not implemented these recommendations. Setting: nursing homes
April 2019	*Management Report: CMS Needs to Address Gaps in Federal Oversight of Nursing Home Abuse Investigations That Persisted in Oregon for at Least 15 Years* (GAO-19-313R)	GAO reviewed CMS oversight of the Oregon state survey agency's investigation of complaints and facility-reported incidents of abuse in nursing homes in Oregon. GAO found that an Oregon agency that was not the survey agency led key nursing home abuse investigations for over 15 years. As a result, until this practice was changed in October 2018, CMS may have missed patterns of abuse and had incomplete information on nursing home quality indicators for both internal CMS purposes and Oregon consumers. GAO made three recommendations including that CMS ensure all state survey agencies are meeting federal requirements for investigating alleged abuse and that the results are shared with CMS. HHS agreed with the recommendations and, as of November 2019, HHS had implemented one of the three recommendations. Setting: nursing homes

Table 1. (Continued)

Date	Title	Description
January 2018	*Medicaid Assisted Living Services: Improved Federal Oversight of Beneficiary Health and Welfare is Needed* (GAO-18-179)	GAO examined state and federal oversight of assisted living services in Medicaid. GAO found oversight of state monitoring of assisted living services by CMS was limited by gaps in state reporting. GAO made three recommendations including that CMS clarify state requirements for reporting program deficiencies and require states to annually report critical incidents. HHS agreed with GAO's recommendations to clarify deficiency reporting and stated that it would consider annual reporting requirements for critical incidents after completing an ongoing review. As of November 2019, HHS had not implemented these recommendations. Setting: assisted living facilities
August 2017	*Medicaid Managed Care: CMS Should Improve Oversight of Access and Quality in States' Long-Term Services and Supports Programs* (GAO-17-632)	GAO reviewed six states' implementation and CMS's oversight of managed long-term services and supports programs. GAO found that these states varied in the extent to which—and how—they monitored concerns about quality and access, and CMS did not always require these states to report the information needed to monitor access and quality. GAO made one recommendation that CMS take steps to identify and obtain information to oversee key aspects of managed long-term services and supports programs' access and quality, including network adequacy, critical incidents, and appeals and grievances. HHS agreed with GAO's recommendation. As of November 2019, HHS had not implemented these recommendations. Setting: nursing homes, assisted living facilities, and others
November 2016	*Elder Abuse: The Extent of Abuse by Guardians Is Unknown, but Some Measures Exist to Help Protect Older Adults* (GAO-17-33)	GAO found that the extent of elder abuse by guardians nationally is unknown due to limited data on key factors. Some efforts are under way to try to collect better data on elder abuse and guardianship at the federal, state, and local levels to support decision making and help prevent and address elder abuse by guardians. GAO did not make any recommendations. Setting: N/A
November 2016	*Medicaid Personal Care Services: CMS Could Do More to Harmonize Requirements across Programs (GAO-17-28)*	GAO reviewed oversight of Medicaid personal care services and found that CMS has taken several steps to improve oversight of states' personal care service programs and harmonize requirements but has not collected required state reports or addressed significant differences in program requirements. GAO made two recommendations including that CMS collect and analyze required state reports on personal care services and take steps to further harmonize federal program requirements, as appropriate, across programs providing these services. HHS concurred with GAO's recommendations. As of November 2019, HHS had implemented one of these two recommendations.

Date	Title	Description
		Setting: In-home
October 2015	*Nursing Home Quality: CMS Should Continue to Improve Data and Oversight* (GAO-16-33)	GAO reviewed trends in nursing home quality data—including data on consumer complaints, deficiencies, staffing levels, and clinical quality measures—and changes in CMS nursing home oversight. GAO found that trends in nursing home quality show mixed results (with data issues complicating the ability to assess quality trends) and that CMS made numerous modifications to its nursing home oversight activities but has not monitored the potential effect of these modifications on nursing home quality oversight. GAO made three recommendations including that CMS implement a clear plan for ongoing auditing of self-reported data and establish a process for monitoring oversight modifications to better assess their effects. HHS agreed with GAO's recommendations. As of November 2019, HHS had implemented one of these three recommendations. Setting: nursing homes
January 2015	*Antipsychotic Drug Use: HHS Has Initiatives to Reduce Use among Older Adults in Nursing Homes, but Should Expand Efforts to Other Settings* (GAO-15-211)	GAO examined psychotropic drug prescribing for older adult nursing home residents and found that about one-third of older adults with dementia, who spent more than 100 days in a nursing home in 2012, were prescribed an antipsychotic, according to data from Medicare's prescription drug program. Among enrollees in this program with dementia living outside of a nursing home that same year, about 14 percent were prescribed an antipsychotic. GAO made one recommendation that HHS expand its outreach and educational efforts aimed at reducing antipsychotic drug use among older adults with dementia to include those residing outside of nursing homes by updating the National Alzheimer's Plan. HHS concurred with GAO's recommendation. As of November 2019, HHS had implemented this recommendation. Setting: nursing homes, assisted living facilities, in-home

Source: GAO. | GAO-20-259T.

APPENDIX II: SEVERITY OF ABUSE DEFICIENCIES CITED IN NURSING HOMES, 2013 THROUGH 2017

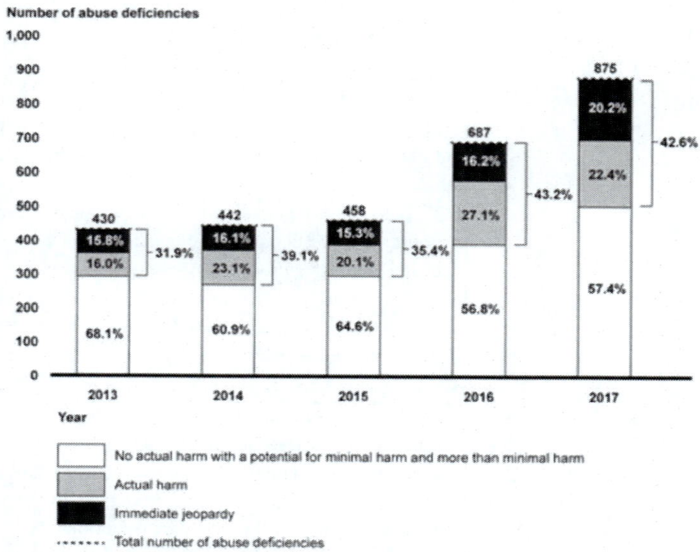

Source: GAO analysis of Centers for Medicare and Medicaid Services (CMS) data. | GAO-20-259T.

Notes: CMS categorizes deficiencies into one of four severity categories based on whether the deficiency constitutes: (1) no actual harm with a potential for minimal harm; (2) no actual harm with a potential for more than minimal harm, but not immediate jeopardy; (3) actual harm that is not immediate jeopardy; or (4) immediate jeopardy to resident health or safety. We combined the first two categories in this figure.

CMS restructured its deficiency code system beginning on November 28, 2017. Due to these coding changes, we did not analyze CMS data cited by surveyors after the implementation of that change.

Percentages may not add to 100 due to rounding.

Figure 1. Severity of Abuse Deficiencies Cited in Nursing Homes, 2013 through 2017.

Appendix III: Examples from a Representative Sample of Nursing Home Abuse Deficiency Narratives, 2016-2017.

Table 2. Examples from a representative sample of nursing home abuse deficiency narratives, 2016-2017

Type(s) of abuse	Type(s) of perpetrator	Narrative details	Scope and severity
Physical abuse	Staff	A nurse aide grabbed a resident by both wrists, causing the resident to fall to the floor and resulting in bruising to the resident's left wrist and left hip.	Isolated scope, immediate jeopardy
Physical and sexual abuse	Resident	Resident 1, who had severe cognitive impairment, kicked another Resident 2, who also had significant cognitive impairment, in the face. Separately, Resident 3 shoved Resident 4 against a door, causing Resident 4 to fall. After being helped up by staff, Resident 4 was hit by Resident 3. The same resident (Resident 3) later slapped a different resident—Resident 5 in the head. Also in the narrative, Resident 6 fondled the breast of Resident 7, who appeared confused by the action.	Isolated scope, actual harm
Sexual and mental/ verbal abuse	Resident and staff	A cognitively impaired resident (Resident 1) with a history of inappropriate sexual behavior grabbed Resident 2 in a sexually inappropriate manner. Resident 1 then grabbed the "private area" of Resident 3. Separately, a nursing home dietary staff member was verbally abusive to a resident (Resident 4), yelling and antagonizing the resident.	Widespread, immediate jeopardy
Sexual abuse	Staff	A nurse aide found a medical technician sexually assaulting a resident in the resident's room. The resident was non-verbal, with severe dementia, and was totally dependent on staff for mobility. The medical technician "begged" the nursing assistant not to tell anyone about witnessing the assault, and the medical technician later told a supervisor they had "had this problem for a while."	Isolated scope, immediate jeopardy

Table 2. (Continued)

Type(s) of abuse	Type(s) of perpetrator	Narrative details	Scope and severity
Mental/ verbal abuse	Other	Resident 1 had an argument with Resident 2. Resident 2's family member arrived and threatened to kick Resident 1 out of her wheelchair if she did not stay away from Resident 2. Resident 1 was deeply concerned and felt frightened every time Resident 2's family member visited and she said that she had a nightmare about the family member.	Isolated scope, no actual harm with a potential for more than minimal harm
Mental/ verbal abuse	Staff	A nurse assistant told a resident to "shut up and (expletive) off" when the resident requested to have their soiled brief changed, and the facility staff member put the resident's call light on the floor under the resident's bed so that the resident would not turn on the call light when they needed care. The state survey agency investigated this complaint, which had not been reported to the facility administrator.	Isolated scope, actual harm

Source: GAO summary of Centers for Medicare & Medicaid Services' (CMS) data. | GAO-20-259T.

Notes: Examples are from our review of a representative sample of abuse deficiency narratives written by state surveyors from 2016 through 2017 that describe abuse. Cited deficiencies are classified into categories according to scope (the number of residents potentially affected) and severity (the potential for or occurrence of harm to residents). The three scope categories include whether the incident was: (1) isolated, (2) constituted a pattern, or (3) widespread. The four severity categories include: (1) no actual harm with a potential for minimal harm; (2) no actual harm with a potential for more than minimal harm, but not immediate jeopardy; (3) actual harm that is not immediate jeopardy; or (4) immediate jeopardy to resident health or safety.

In: Nursing Homes and Elder Abuse
Editor: Joshua Newland
ISBN: 978-1-53617-974-3
© 2020 Nova Science Publishers, Inc.

Chapter 4

ELDER ABUSE: FEDERAL REQUIREMENTS FOR OVERSIGHT IN NURSING HOMES AND ASSISTED LIVING FACILITIES DIFFER*

United States Government Accountability Office

ABBREVIATIONS

APS	Adult Protective Services
CMS	Centers for Medicare & Medicaid Services
HCBS	home and community-based services
HHS	Department of Health and Human Services
HHS-OIG	Department of Health and Human Services' Office of Inspector General
SSA	Social Security Act

* This is an edited, reformatted and augmented version of United States Government Accountability Office; Report to Congressional Requesters, Publication No. GAO-19-599, dated August 2019.

Why GAO Did This Study

The federal government and states share responsibility for the health and welfare of about 1.5 million individuals— most of them vulnerable older adults— receiving long-term care in nursing homes and assisted living facilities covered by Medicare and Medicaid. For nursing homes, which provide skilled nursing care, federal law defines applicable quality standards and CMS provides guidance for nursing homes and the state survey agencies to help protect residents from elder abuse. For assisted living facilities, which provide assistance with activities of daily living in a residential setting, CMS defines the framework states must establish to oversee these facilities if covered under Medicaid. This includes requiring states to demonstrate to CMS that they are assuring quality including the obligation to protect against elder abuse.

GAO was asked to review federal oversight of elder abuse reporting, investigation, and law enforcement notification in both nursing homes and assisted living facilities. In this report, GAO describes federal requirements for reporting, investigating, and notifying law enforcement about elder abuse in both types of facilities. GAO reviewed relevant laws and regulations and agency guidance, and interviewed CMS and state officials from three states selected for variation in HCBS waiver program size and geography. GAO also interviewed representatives from national stakeholder groups representing consumers, facilities, Medicaid directors, and abuse investigators. In comments on this report, HHS highlighted the distinct oversight frameworks for the two settings and noted that CMS is undertaking efforts to strengthen oversight.

What GAO Found

The Centers for Medicare & Medicaid Services (CMS) oversees the Medicare and Medicaid programs and is responsible for safeguarding the health and welfare of beneficiaries living in nursing homes and assisted living facilities. This includes safeguarding older residents from abuse—

referred to as elder abuse. CMS delegates responsibility for overseeing this issue to state survey agencies, which are responsible for overseeing nursing homes. When assisted living facilities provide services to Medicaid beneficiaries, they are indirectly subject to CMS oversight through the agency's oversight of state Medicaid agencies.

	Nursing homes		Assisted living facilities	
Federal requirement	Homes	State survey agencies	Facilities	State Medicaid agencies
Report incident to oversight agency[a]	●	●	○	⊗
Investigate incidents	●	●	○	⊗
Notify law enforcement of incidents	●[b]	●	○	○

● Required to take specified actions

⊗ Required to establish state- or facility-level policy

○ Not required to take specific action or establish policy

Source: GAO analysis of federal regulations and guidance. | GAO-19-599

Note: This table reflects federal requirements applicable to services provided in assisted living facilities under section 1915(c) of the Social Security Act.

[a] Nursing homes are required to ensure that incidents are reported to state survey agencies. State survey agencies are required to report certain incidents to CMS and state Medicaid agencies are required to report incidents to CMS according to the state's individual 1915(c) waiver agreement.

[b] Federal law requires certain covered individuals at the nursing homes to immediately report to law enforcement in addition to the state survey agency if there is a reasonable suspicion that a crime has occurred. See 42 U.S.C. § 1320b-25(b).

Federal Requirements for Facilities and State Agencies to Conduct Elder Abuse Incident Reporting, Investigation, and Law Enforcement Notification

GAO found that there are specific federal requirements for nursing homes and state survey agencies for reporting, investigating, and notifying law enforcement about elder abuse in nursing homes. (See table below). For example, state survey agencies must prioritize reports of elder abuse in nursing homes based on CMS's specified criteria and investigate within specific time frames. In contrast, there are no similar federal requirements for assisted living facilities— which are licensed and regulated by states. Instead, CMS requires state Medicaid agencies to develop policies to ensure the reporting and investigation of elder abuse in assisted living facilities. For example, CMS requires that state Medicaid agencies establish their own policies and standards for prioritizing reports when investigating incidents in assisted living facilities. Officials from the three selected states in GAO's review said they apply certain federal nursing home requirements and investigation time frames for assisted living facilities when overseeing elder abuse.

August 19, 2019

The Honorable Susan M. Collins
Chairman
Special Committee on Aging
United States Senate

The Honorable Amy Klobuchar
Ranking Member
Committee on Rules and Administration
United States Senate

The federal government and states share responsibility for the health and welfare of approximately 1.5 million individuals—most of them older adults—receiving care in long-term care facilities financed by Medicare and Medicaid, the federal health care programs for the elderly and low-income and medically needy individuals, respectively.[1] These facilities include nursing homes, which provide skilled nursing and rehabilitative care to elderly and disabled individuals, and assisted living facilities, which provide a residential alternative to nursing home care for individuals who

[1] Medicare, the federal health insurance program for people age 65 and older, individuals under age 65 with certain disabilities, and individuals diagnosed with end-stage renal disease, covers some short-term skilled nursing and rehabilitative care for beneficiaries following an acute care hospital stay. Medicaid, a joint federal-state health program for low-income and medically needy individuals, is the nation's primary payer of long-term services and supports for children and adults with disabilities and aged individuals.

may prefer to live independently but need assistance with daily activities.[2] Residents of both types of facilities often have physical and cognitive limitations that can make them particularly vulnerable to abuse. Abuse, which can be committed by facility staff, residents, or others, is a serious occurrence and could result in potentially devastating consequences for the victim, including lasting mental anguish, serious injury, or death. While abuse is a concern for both elderly and nonelderly individuals in long-term care facilities, this report focuses on federal oversight to protect elderly residents of these facilities from abuse, more specifically known as elder abuse.[3]

Federal law mandates that nursing homes receiving Medicare and Medicaid payment must ensure that residents are free from abuse, neglect, and exploitation.[4] Nursing homes must meet a comprehensive set of federal statutory and regulatory requirements in order to receive such payments. The Centers for Medicare & Medicaid Services (CMS)— the agency within the Department of Health and Human Services (HHS) that oversees the Medicare and Medicaid programs—is responsible for implementing these requirements. In 2016, nursing homes provided care to approximately 1.4 million individuals.[5]

In contrast to nursing homes, assisted living facilities are primarily overseen at the state level through state licensing and regulatory requirements. States that provide Medicaid coverage of assisted living facility services for older adults typically do so through a home and

---

[2] Depending on the state, assisted living services—including services such as bathing, dressing, and toileting—can be regulated separately from the facility that provides residential services. However, for the purposes of this report we refer to the assisted living services as those provided in assisted living facilities and do not include services provided in an individual's home or family member's home.

[3] We have issued several reports on different types of elder abuse and across different settings. For example, in a June 2019 report, we examined the Department of Justice's efforts to address crimes against older adults. See GAO, *Elder Justice: Goals and Outcome Measures Would Provide DOJ with Clear Direction and a Means to Assess Its Efforts,* GAO-19-365 (Washington, DC: June 7, 2019). We have also issued reports focused on the financial exploitation of elders, a topic not addressed in this report. Information on these reports is available on our Key Issues page, https://www.gao.gov/key_issues/elder_abuse/issue_summary?from=topics#t=1

[4] This report addresses these rights as they pertain to individuals age 65 or older and refers to the violation of these rights as "elder abuse."

[5] Of the 1.4 million nursing home residents, 83.5 percent—or 1.1 million—are over the age of 65.

community-based service (HCBS) waiver under section 1915(c) of the Social Security Act (SSA).[6] Under these waivers, states are responsible for developing adequate standards to protect the health and safety of beneficiaries receiving services under the waiver and must demonstrate to CMS that these standards are met. In 2016, Medicaid covered assisted living facility services for an estimated 125,000 elderly beneficiaries.[7]

In recent reports, we have found that improved federal oversight of the health and welfare of residents is needed in both nursing homes and assisted living facilities.[8] For example, as we reported in our June 2019 report, we found that the incidence of abuse in nursing homes as identified by state survey agencies increased between 2013 and 2017, and in January 2018, we found that little is known about the incidence of abuse in assisted

---

[6] Section1915(c) of the Social Security Act (SSA), authorizes the Secretary of Health and Human Services (HHS) to waive otherwise applicable requirements that states offering HCBS offer comparable benefits statewide, offer comparable program benefits to all eligible beneficiaries, and use a single standard to determine income and resources for purposes of eligibility. For purposes of this report, references to "HCBS waiver" programs refer to HCBS offered under section 1915(c). States most commonly use section 1915(c) waivers to cover assisted living services under their Medicaid programs, but Medicaid coverage may also be provided under the state's Medicaid plan or through Medicaid demonstrations authorized under section 1115 of the SSA, which allows the Secretary of HHS to waive certain federal Medicaid requirements and allow costs that would not otherwise be eligible for federal matching funds for experimental, pilot, or demonstration projects that, in the Secretary's judgment, are likely to assist in promoting Medicaid objectives. Among these different Medicaid authorities, as we previously reported, section 1915(c) waivers have the most federal health and safety requirements. See GAO, *Medicaid Personal Care Services: CMS Could Do More to Harmonize Requirements across Programs,* GAO-17-28, (Washington D.C.: Nov. 23, 2016).

[7] In 2016, approximately 757,941 elderly individuals received services in residential care communities specializing in services for the elderly, such as assisted living facilities. Of those, 16.5 percent—approximately 125,000 individuals—reported using Medicaid as a payer source. Harris-Kojetin L, Sengupta M, Lendon JP, Rome V, Valverde R, Caffrey C. Long-term care providers and services users in the United States, 2015–2016. National Center for Health Statistics. Vital Health Stat 3(43). 2019.

[8] See GAO, *Nursing Homes: Improved Oversight Needed to Protect Residents from Abuse*, GAO-19-433 (Washington, D.C.: June 13, 2019); *Nursing Home Quality: CMS Should Continue to Improve Data and Oversight*, GAO-16-33 (Washington, D.C.: Oct. 30, 2015); *Medicaid Personal Care Services: CMS Could Do More to Harmonize Requirements across Programs*, GAO-17-28 (Washington, D.C.: Nov. 23, 2016); *Medicaid Managed Care: CMS Should Improve Oversight of Access and Quality in States' Long- Term Services and Supports Programs*, GAO-17-632 (Washington, D.C.: Aug. 14, 2017); *and Medicaid Assisted Living Services: Improved Federal Oversight of Beneficiary Health and Welfare Is Needed*, GAO-18-179 (Washington, D.C.: Jan. 5, 2018).

living facilities.[9] In CMS's oversight of both settings, we found a lack of clear federal guidance on reporting and consequently, a lack of key information necessary for monitoring incidents that may cause harm to a beneficiary's health or welfare, such as abuse. Additionally, the HHS Office of Inspector General (HHS-OIG) and state auditors have also examined how elder abuse is reported and investigated and recommended improvements at both the federal and state level.

You asked us to review federal oversight of the reporting, investigation, and notification of law enforcement about elder abuse in nursing homes and assisted living facilities. In this report, we describe federal requirements for reporting, investigating, and notifying law enforcement about elder abuse in both types of facilities. In appendix I, we provide information on efforts by three selected states to meet federal requirements for reporting, investigating, and notifying law enforcement about elder abuse in assisted living facilities. In appendix II, we provide summary information from other federal and state audits of elder abuse reporting and investigation. Further, throughout this report we note our past work on this topic.

To describe federal requirements for reporting, investigating, and notifying law enforcement about elder abuse in nursing homes and assisted living facilities, we reviewed relevant statutes and regulations and CMS guidance, including the State Operations Manual and HCBS waiver guidance and interviewed CMS officials regarding the agency's oversight of the requirements. We selected a non-generalizable sample of three states—Connecticut, Oklahoma, and South Dakota—that have implemented HCBS waivers and vary in HCBS waiver program size and geography.[10] In each state, we reviewed their waiver agreements and spoke with officials from the state survey agency, state Medicaid agency, and the state agency responsible for licensing assisted living facilities and

---

[9] GAO-19-433; GAO-18-179.

[10] For each of our selected states, we reviewed publicly available Centers for Disease Control & Prevention data on long-term care providers and services users to obtain state- level data on the number of assisted living facilities, beds, and residents receiving care financed by Medicaid.

investigating complaints.[11] We also interviewed CMS officials, including regional office officials, about their oversight of state survey agencies and HCBS waivers in our selected states. We interviewed representatives from national stakeholder groups representing consumers, facilities, Medicaid directors, and investigators to obtain their perspectives on elder abuse in nursing homes and assisted living facilities. We also reviewed related audits issued by the HHS-OIG and state auditors between 2014 and 2018 related to reporting and investigating elder abuse in nursing homes and assisted living facilities and included them with a discussion of related GAO reports.

We conducted this performance audit from August 2018 to August 2019 in accordance with generally accepted government auditing standards. Those standards require that we plan and perform the audit to obtain sufficient, appropriate evidence to provide a reasonable basis for our findings and conclusions based on our audit objectives. We believe that the evidence obtained provides a reasonable basis for our findings and conclusions based on our audit objectives.

BACKGROUND

Care Provided in Nursing Homes and Assisted Living Facilities

Nursing homes and assisted living facilities provide important long-term care to vulnerable individuals in institutional or residential settings. Specifically, nursing homes provide care to elderly and disabled individuals, many of whom have physical and cognitive limitations requiring skilled nursing care. Assisted living facilities provide a residential alternative to nursing home care for individuals who prefer to live independently but need assistance to maintain their independence. Like nursing homes, they may provide residents with a variety of services

[11] To oversee nursing homes, CMS enters into agreements with agencies in each state government—known as state survey agencies—and CMS regional offices oversee the work done by the state survey agencies. Survey agencies are frequently housed in the health services department of state governments and may have different names in different states.

to assist with activities of daily living, such as bathing and dressing, but the facilities are generally not licensed to provide 24-hour skilled nursing care and typically offer a more limited range of medical care. As we reported in our January 2018 report on CMS's oversight of assisted living facilities under the Medicaid program, the demand for assisted living services, which offer the benefit of community living, is expected to increase as a result of the aging of the nation's population, increased life expectancy, and older adults' desire to remain in the community.[12] Additionally, the cost of nursing home care for an individual generally exceeds the cost of assisted living facility services, further incentivizing a shift among consumers and payers to assisted living for elderly individuals, including those with increasingly complex health needs who would otherwise need nursing home care.[13]

Long-Term Care Facility Oversight

Oversight of nursing homes is a shared federal-state responsibility. Federal law imposes both a comprehensive set of quality standards that nursing homes must meet to participate in the Medicare and Medicaid programs, and federal and state oversight responsibilities to enforce these standards. CMS, which is charged with implementing these standards and conducting federal oversight, contracts with state survey agencies to perform both routine inspections—known as standard surveys—and conduct investigations of elder abuse incidents, including complaints and facility-reported incidents.[14] CMS provides guidance implementing

---

[12] See GAO, *Medicaid Assisted Living Services: Improved Federal Oversight of Beneficiary Health and Welfare Is Needed,* GAO-18-179 (Washington, D.C.: Jan. 5, 2018).

[13] Genworth Financial, Inc. *Cost of Care Survey* (Richmond, VA. October 2018). This industry study found that the median national cost for a year of nursing home care in a semi-private room was $89,297 per year, compared to a national median cost of $48,000 a year for care in an assisted living facility.

[14] Standard surveys are a comprehensive on-site evaluation of compliance with federal quality standards, during which surveyors must identify and report any deficiencies, which are classified by the potential for or occurrence of harm to residents. In addition, state survey agencies can receive information about elder abuse incidents through complaints and facility reported incidents. Complaints can be submitted verbally or in writing from

statutory and regulatory requirements to protect residents from elder abuse in its State Operations Manual, which specifies requirements for reporting, investigating, and notifying law enforcement about elder abuse in nursing homes. CMS regional offices monitor state compliance with federal requirements for nursing home oversight.

Generally, states establish their own oversight requirements for assisted living facilities. These facilities are largely overseen by state agencies within, for example, the state health or aging departments; however, when assisted living facilities provide services to Medicaid beneficiaries, they are also indirectly subject to CMS oversight through the agency's oversight of state Medicaid agencies. As we have previously reported, states can provide Medicaid coverage for assisted living services under multiple authorities, but most commonly states use an HCBS waiver under section 1915(c) of the SSA.[15] Under these waivers, CMS requires states to develop a quality assurance system that monitors beneficiary health and welfare—including tracking and responding to incidents that may cause harm to a beneficiary's health and welfare, such as elder abuse.[16] States must demonstrate to CMS that they are meeting these quality assurance obligations in their waiver renewal reports, typically submitted about 2 years before an HCBS waiver is scheduled to end.[17] States must also report summary information annually to CMS on any

residents, their family members, health care providers, state agencies, and anonymous sources. Facilities also report incidents to the state survey agency to be assessed for investigation.

[15] HCBS waivers serve beneficiaries who are eligible for an institutional level of care; that is, beneficiaries must have needs that rise to the level of care usually provided in a nursing home. HCBS waivers are generally approved for an initial 3-year period and can be renewed, subject to HHS approval, for subsequent 5-year waiver periods.

[16] These incidents are commonly referred to as critical incidents. As we previously reported, although states vary in how they define critical incidents, the 48 states that covered assisted living through their HCBS waivers in 2014 all cited physical, emotional, and sexual abuse as a critical incident. See GAO-18-179. Among other things, we recommended that CMS establish standard reporting requirements for states to report key information on critical incidents. CMS neither agreed nor disagreed with our recommendation and as of June 2019, has yet to take action.

[17] In renewal reports, states are required to report to CMS on performance indicators, selected at the state's discretion, that demonstrate compliance with more specific assurances. Specifically, states must identify measures they will use to monitor the specified assurances for beneficiary health and welfare and submit evidentiary reports to CMS demonstrating that the state has met these assurances before a waiver can be renewed.

health and welfare deficiencies occurring under their HCBS waivers. CMS regional offices oversee state compliance with waiver requirements.

In addition to state survey agencies, state Medicaid agencies, and the agencies that license and regulate assisted living facilities, there are other entities charged with protecting nursing home and assisted living facility residents from elder abuse. These agencies' roles and missions can vary by state. For example, Adult Protective Services (APS) programs in each state are generally responsible for identifying, investigating, resolving, and preventing abuse of older adults, and such programs may investigate complaints of elder abuse in nursing homes and assisted living facilities.[18] Additionally, Medicaid Fraud Control Units and local law enforcement can also play a role in investigating elder abuse. Consequently, incident management may be coordinated among multiple separate agencies.[19]

FEDERAL REQUIREMENTS SPECIFY ELDER ABUSE REPORTING, INVESTIGATION, AND NOTIFICATION IN NURSING HOMES AND DIRECT STATES TO ESTABLISH ASSISTED LIVING FACILITY REQUIREMENTS

Federal requirements include those for nursing homes and state survey agencies specific to reporting, investigating, and notifying law enforcement of elder abuse in nursing homes. For example, federal requirements specify the time frames within which nursing homes must report alleged elder abuse to state survey agencies and, similarly, specify time frames for state survey agencies to report elder abuse to CMS. In contrast, there are no similar requirements for assisted living facilities and, instead, states must establish their own policies to ensure the reporting and investigation of elder abuse in assisted living facilities covered by Medicaid.

---

[18] In some states, APS is not responsible for investigating elder abuse in nursing homes.

[19] As we reported in GAO-19-433, having multiple agencies—such as the state survey agency, adult protective services, local law enforcement—involved in investigations, can create challenges for coordinating investigations.

	Nursing homes		Assisted living facilities	
Federal requirement	Homes	State survey agencies	Facilities	State Medicaid agencies
Reporting				
Report incidents to oversight agency according to specified time frames[a]	●	●	○	○
Establish a policy for reporting incidents to oversight agency	●	○[b]	○	●
Investigation				
Investigate incidents according to specified time frames	●	●	○	○
Establish a policy for investigating incidents	●	●	○	●
Law Enforcement Notification				
Notify law enforcement according to specified time frames or circumstances	●[c]	●[d]	○	○
Establish a policy for notifying law enforcement	●	○[b]	○	○

● Required
○ Not required

Source: GAO analysis of federal regulations and guidance. | GAO-19-599

Note: This figure reflects federal requirements applicable to services provided in assisted living facilities to participants in a home and community-based waiver authorized under section 1915(c) of the Social Security Act. Elder abuse incidents include incidents reported by nursing homes or assisted living facilities and complaints reported by the alleged victim or other concerned individual. Certain requirements only apply to facility reported incidents, or apply to these incidents differently than complaints, as noted in the figure. States may choose to impose similar or additional requirements on assisted living facilities providing services under section 1915(c) waivers. See app. I for a summary of selected states' requirements for reporting, investigating, and notifying law enforcement about elder abuse in assisted living facilities.

[a] Nursing homes are required to ensure that incidents are reported to state survey agencies. State survey agencies must report to CMS all complaints gathered as part of the agency's federal survey and certification responsibilities but do not have to report facility-reported incidents that do not require an on-site investigation. State Medicaid agencies are not required to report individual incidents of elder abuse that occur under the HCBS waiver until they have been substantiated. State Medicaid agencies may also share summary data about elder abuse with CMS through required annual reports or as part of the state's waiver renewal process.

[b] CMS defines policies for the state survey agencies in these areas.

[c] Federal law requires certain covered individuals at the nursing homes to immediately report to law enforcement in addition to the state survey agency if there is a reasonable suspicion that a crime has occurred. See 42 U.S.C. § 1320b-25(b). These covered individuals include nursing home owners, operators, and employees, among others. CMS requires nursing homes to ensure compliance with this provision.

[d] CMS requires state survey agencies to notify law enforcement of substantiated findings of abuse; however, it does not specify time frames for notification. As GAO noted in GAO-19-433, this can result in significant delay and we recommended that CMS require state survey agencies to immediately notify law enforcement if they have a reasonable suspicion that a crime against a resident has occurred.

Figure 1. Federal Requirements for Elder Abuse Incident Reporting, Investigation, and Law Enforcement Notification.

(See Figure 1 for federal requirements for reporting, investigating, and notifying law enforcement about elder abuse in nursing homes and assisted living facilities.) As illustrated in Figure 1, there are key differences between federal requirements for reporting, investigating, and notifying law enforcement about elder abuse occurring in nursing homes compared to assisted living facilities. CMS officials told us that the difference in requirements between nursing homes and assisted living facilities reflects the different regulatory relationship between the agency and the two facility types. According to CMS officials, CMS has direct regulatory authority over nursing homes, but does not have direct authority over assisted living facilities. As noted, states are largely responsible for establishing their own policies for overseeing the reporting and investigation of abuse in assisted living facilities. (See app. I for profiles of selected states with HCBS waivers regarding elder abuse reporting, investigating, and notification.) Differences in federal requirements include the following:

Reporting

Federal law and CMS policy define specific time frames for nursing home staff and state survey agencies to report incidents of abuse that occur in nursing homes, respectively, and CMS requires states to establish their own reporting time frames for assisted living facilities serving HCBS waiver participants.[20] Nursing homes must ensure that allegations of elder abuse are reported to the state survey agency immediately, but no later than 2 hours after the allegation is made if the incident involves serious bodily injuries and within 24 hours if it does not. In addition, state survey agencies must report to CMS all complaints and certain facility-reported incidents of abuse through a computer-based complaint and incident tracking system and immediately alert CMS regional offices when an

[20] Federal law requires certain covered individuals at the nursing homes to immediately report to law enforcement in addition to the state survey agency if there is a reasonable suspicion that a crime has occurred. See 42 U.S.C. § 1320b-25(b). These covered individuals include nursing home owners, operators, and employees, among others.

especially significant or sensitive incident occurs that attracts public or broad media attention.[21] In contrast, CMS requires state Medicaid agencies that pay for care in assisted living facilities through HCBS waivers to establish their own required time frames for reporting incidents.[22] Consequently, reporting time frames and processes for assisted living facilities can vary by state. For example, Connecticut requires incidents to be reported to the state Medicaid agency and Adult Protective Services within 2 business days, while Oklahoma requires that initial incident reports are submitted within 1 business day.

Investigation

CMS prescribes investigation time frames and priority categories for incidents occurring in nursing homes and requires states to establish their own time frames and priority categories for incidents in assisted living facilities. CMS requires state survey agencies to assess reports of elder abuse in nursing homes and assign a priority investigation status based on the seriousness of the allegations. The required investigation time frames are tied to the priority status. For example, if the allegation indicates that there continues to be an immediate risk of serious injury, harm, impairment, or death of a resident unless immediate corrective action is taken, the survey agency must initiate an onsite investigation within 2 business days of receiving the report.[23]

---

[21] State survey agencies are required to enter into CMS's tracking system all complaint information gathered as part of the agency's federal survey and certification responsibilities, as well as all facility-reported incidents that require a federal onsite survey.

[22] Federal law requires states to report annually to CMS summary information about health and welfare deficiencies—such as incidents of abuse—found through state monitoring of their HCBS program. However, as we previously reported, CMS gives states wide latitude for determining what to include in these reports and does not require states to regularly provide CMS information on critical incidents. See GAO-18-179.

[23] CMS requires survey agencies to assign incidents to one of four prioritization categories and adhere to the following associated processes for initiating investigations: Immediate Jeopardy requires the agency to start onsite investigation within 2 business days of receipt; Non-Immediate Jeopardy High Priority requires onsite investigation within 10 days of prioritization; Non-Immediate Jeopardy Medium requires onsite survey to be scheduled (no

Family or Legal Guardian Notification

Although the Centers for Medicare & Medicaid Services (CMS) requires facilities to notify a resident's representative of a deterioration in the resident's condition, CMS does not require nursing homes, assisted living facilities, state survey agencies, or state Medicaid agencies to notify a victim's family or legal guardian of alleged elder abuse. However, CMS's guidance for nursing homes notes the importance of family or legal guardian notification. Specifically, CMS guidance requires facilities to take actions to prevent further harm from occurring to a victim of alleged elder abuse and cites law enforcement notification, as well as family or legal guardian notification as examples of protective measures facilities may take to comply with that requirement. In addition, CMS requires states to develop a policy for notifying participants, family, or legal guardians of the findings of any critical incident investigations under its home and community-based services waiver program. CMS officials told us family or legal guardian notification is generally a state responsibility, and state officials told us that it is largely a facility responsibility governed by the facility's policies. Some states include family or guardian notification requirements in state guidance on mandatory reporting of elder abuse. In interviews with stakeholders representing consumers and elder abuse investigators we learned that family notification can both help but also pose some privacy challenges.

Source: GAO analysis | GAO-19-599

CMS also requires nursing homes to have written policies and procedures for conducting internal investigations of suspected elder abuse and to submit findings from these investigations to the state survey agency within 5 business days of the incident. In contrast, CMS does not prescribe investigation time frames or define priorities for incidents occurring in assisted living facilities; instead, CMS requires that state Medicaid agencies with HCBS waivers establish their own policies for prioritizing

---

time frame specified); Non- Immediate Jeopardy Low requires investigation during the next survey.

reports of abuse and initiating investigations in assisted living facilities.[24] Consequently, investigation time frames and prioritization can vary by state. For example, Connecticut does not specify a process for prioritizing incident investigations in its HCBS waiver, but officials told us the state requires the Medicaid program to initiate an investigation immediately; whereas South Dakota requires face-to- face contact with a victim within 24 hours if the incident is life or health-threatening.

Law Enforcement Notification

Although federal law requires nursing homes to establish policies for ensuring that law enforcement is notified of elder abuse that occurs in their facilities, and CMS policy requires state survey agencies to notify law enforcement of substantiated findings of elder abuse that occur in nursing homes, these actions are not required when a similar incident occurs in an assisted living facility. Furthermore, CMS also does not require state Medicaid agencies to establish their own law enforcement notification requirements for assisted living facilities as part of the state's HCBS waiver agreements. CMS and state officials told us that, generally, state agencies coordinate with law enforcement regardless of where the abuse occurs. Some states also require law enforcement notification as part of their state mandatory reporter laws.[25] (See app. I for descriptions of selected state mandatory reporter laws.) For example, Connecticut requires Medicaid waiver program staff members to inform law enforcement of all suspected crimes, including abuse. Both GAO and HHS-OIG have identified, among other things, gaps in notifying law enforcement about

---

[24] As we previously reported in January 2018, state Medicaid agencies' definitions of incidents that facilities must report to the state vary and therefore, some incidents that could be considered elder abuse, such as a resident's unauthorized seclusion or restraint by a provider, may not routinely be reported to the state Medicaid agency in some states. See GAO, *Medicaid Assisted Living Services: Improved Federal Oversight of Beneficiary Health and Welfare Is Needed,* GAO-18-179 (Washington, D.C.: Jan. 5, 2018).

[25] Almost all states have mandated reporter laws for elder abuse that require various identified health care providers and facility staff, among others, to report suspected elder abuse to state oversight agencies or law enforcement.

abuse in nursing homes and recommended that CMS make changes to help ensure that nursing homes and state survey agencies notify law enforcement.[26]

In the course of our review, we found states may align certain requirements for investigating, reporting, and notifying law enforcement about elder abuse in assisted living facilities with federal requirements for nursing homes. Officials from all three selected states in our review told us they apply certain federal nursing home requirements and time frames to assisted living facilities when overseeing reports and investigations of alleged elder abuse. For example, officials from Oklahoma and South Dakota told us they align or are in the process of aligning time frames within which assisted living facilities are required to report incidents of elder abuse to state authorities with the time frames federally required for nursing homes, and said that alignment reduces confusion, especially among facilities that offer both types of residential care.

Given its attenuated role in overseeing the reporting, investigation, and law enforcement notification of elder abuse in assisted living facilities, CMS officials told us the agency is taking steps to gather and disseminate best practices to help states better manage their response to elder abuse incidents in assisted living facilities. Specifically, officials told us that CMS has initiated an effort to more closely examine how states operate their incident management systems, which are used to track reports and investigations of elder abuse in assisted living facilities covered by their HCBS waivers.[27] In May 2018, CMS surveyed states requesting information on how those states operate an incident management system for their HCBS waiver programs to track reports and investigations of

---

[26] In June 2019 GAO reported that because there is no federal requirement for state survey agencies to notify law enforcement until the state survey agency has substantiated a suspected crime, there were delays in referring suspected crime to law enforcement, and recommended that CMS require state survey agencies to immediately refer suspected crime to law enforcement. See GAO-19-433. See app. II for information on HHS-OIG and state auditor reports on the reporting and investigation of elder abuse.

[27] States use the information in these systems, in part, to provide their quality assurances to CMS as part of its HCBS waiver oversight.

elder abuse.[28] CMS officials said they will take information learned through the survey as well as through on-site reviews that the agency has been conducting in five states since June 2019, to develop best practices and technical guidance on collecting and reporting critical incidents.

AGENCY COMMENTS

We provided a draft of this report to HHS for review and comment. HHS noted that federal oversight of nursing homes and assisted living facilities is not directly comparable given the differences between HHS's statutory authority to oversee both facility types. HHS noted that although CMS's oversight of assisted living facilities is more limited, CMS works in partnership with states—through providing guidance, technical support, training, and oversight of states' quality reporting—to ensure the safety of Medicaid beneficiaries in assisted living facilities. We recognize that CMS is operating in different statutory frameworks with respect to both nursing homes and assisted living facilities, and we have noted the distinction in our report. HHS further noted that CMS is undertaking efforts to strengthen federal oversight of nursing homes and states with HCBS programs, including through addressing our past recommendations. HHS comments are reproduced in appendix III. HHS also provided technical comments, which were incorporated as appropriate. As agreed with your offices, unless you publicly announce the contents of this report earlier, we plan no further distribution until 30 days from the report date. At that time, we will send copies of this report to the Secretary of Health and Human Services, appropriate congressional committees, and other interested parties.

John E. Dicken
Director, Health Care

[28] CMS fielded a pilot survey of seven states in May 2018. Among other things, the pilot survey found variation among the states' required time frames for reporting incidents and that most waiver programs do not notify beneficiaries about a provider's involvement in prior incidents of elder abuse.

APPENDIX I: SUMMARY OF SELECTED STATES' REQUIREMENTS FOR REPORTING, INVESTIGATING, AND NOTIFYING LAW ENFORCEMENT ABOUT ELDER ABUSE IN ASSISTED LIVING FACILITIES

We reviewed state-level requirements for reporting, investigating, and notifying law enforcement about elder abuse in three selected states that cover services in assisted living facilities under their Home and Community-based Services (HCBS) waivers—Connecticut, Oklahoma, and South Dakota. These states are collectively responsible for safeguarding as many as 16,800 assisted living residents—2,751 of whom are covered by Medicaid—from elder abuse. All three states have mandatory reporting requirements that typically require various identified health care providers and facility staff to report suspected elder abuse to adult protective services or law enforcement, regardless of the setting in which the victim was abused or whether the victim is an HCBS waiver participant who would be protected under the Centers for Medicare & Medicaid Services (CMS) program requirements.[29] Further, the states developed guidance for their HCBS programs that establishes additional reporting, investigation, and notification requirements—beyond their mandatory reporting law requirements—that caregivers, facilities, program staff, and state agencies must follow in response to incidents that occur to residents receiving services under Medicaid waiver programs. Selected information about assisted living facilities and state-level requirements for each of the three states is summarized in Figures 2 through 4

[29] We identified these states' mandatory reporting laws using resources available through the Department of Justice Elder Justice Initiative and confirmed this information with the states. The Elder Justice Initiative is the Department of Justice's program to support and coordinate enforcement and programmatic efforts to combat elder abuse, neglect, and financial fraud and scams that target seniors.

Numbers of Assisted Living Facilities, Licensed Beds, and Residents Financed by Medicaid Dollars, 2014			
State	**Number of facilities**	**Number of beds**	**Number of residents financed by Medicaid**
Connecticut	60	1,700	1,261[a]

Selected Mandatory Reporter Requirements

Reporting

Reporters, including nurse's aides or facility administrators, with reasonable cause to believe that a long-term care resident has been abused, must report the information to Connecticut's Department of Social Services' Adult Protective Services (APS) program within 72 hours.[b]

Investigating

Upon receipt of a report, APS determines whether there are reasonable grounds for an investigation. If no grounds, then that determination must be made within 5 working days and reported to the complainant. If an investigation is warranted, it must begin within 10 working days and completed within 15 working days of receiving the report.

Notifying

Incidents meeting the state's legal standard of abuse must be reported to law enforcement. APS must notify a guardian within 24 hours unless the guardian is suspected of perpetrating the abuse.

Home and Community-based Services (HCBS) Waiver Program Requirements

CMS waiver requires states specify	Connecticut's HCBS program requirements
Reporting	
Which types of incidents must be reported	Allegations of abuse, neglect, or exploitation, along with other incidents such as untimely death or unplanned hospitalization must be reported.
Who must report incidents	All members of the participant's care planning team, support staff, and service agency officials are required to report incidents.
Time frames for reporting incidents	Reports must be made within two business days.
To whom reports are submitted	Reports must be made to the Medicaid program's quality assurance unit and, in cases involving abuse, neglect, or exploitation, to APS and law enforcement.
Investigating	
Who is responsible for assessing incidents and conducting investigations	A dedicated Medicaid program quality assurance unit conducts the initial assessment.
How incidents are assessed	Departments involved with HCBS waivers initiate investigations; specific manner of follow-up is determined by the nature of the allegation.
Time frame for conducting and completing an investigation	No time frames specified in the waiver agreement
Notifying	
Process for informing the participant, or the participant's family or legal representative and other relevant parties, of the investigation results	Law enforcement: suspected crimes must be reported to law enforcement. Participant: must receive a copy of critical incident report. Family or legal representative: must receive a copy of critical incident report.[c] Licensing and regulatory agency: no notification requirements specified in the waiver agreement.

Source: GAO analysis of the Centers for Diseases Control & Prevention data and the Centers for Medicare & Medicaid Services (CMS) HCBS waiver technical guidance and Connecticut's waiver agreement. | GAO-19-599

[a] Connecticut also provides financial assistance to assisted living residents separate from federal-state Medicaid funding. Medicaid made payments for 79 percent of assisted living residents in Connecticut in 2014.

[b] Connecticut's APS program that serves individuals age 60 or older is called Protective Services for the Elderly.

[c] According to Connecticut's waiver agreement, incidents must be reported to a participant's conservator, or court appointed representative, who may or may not be a family member.

Figure 2. Connecticut State Profile.

Numbers of Assisted Living Facilities, Licensed Beds, and Residents Financed by Medicaid Dollars, 2014

State	Number of facilities	Number of beds	Number of residents financed by Medicaid
Oklahoma	200	10,500	458[a]

Selected Mandatory Reporter Requirements

Reporting

Reporters, including assisted living facility staff, must report instances of abuse, neglect, or exploitation to Oklahoma's Department of Human Services', Adult Protective Services (APS) program or local law enforcement, as soon as they are aware of the situation.

Investigating

While investigations must be prompt, no specific time frames for initiating or completing APS investigations are noted in requirements.

Notifying

APS must notify law enforcement of the agency's investigation. In addition, APS must notify the victim's caretaker, legal guardian, and next of kin of the initiation of an investigation, and whether there has been a finding of abuse, neglect, or exploitation.

Home and Community-based Services (HCBS) Waiver Program Requirements

CMS waiver requires states specify	Oklahoma's HCBS program requirements
Reporting	
Which types of incidents must be reported	Allegations of sexual and physical abuse, neglect, or exploitation, along with other incidents such as injuries requiring medical attention, or unexpected death must be reported.
Who must report incidents	Waiver program contracted care providers are required to report incidents.
Time frames for reporting incidents	Providers must submit initial reports within 1 business day.
To whom reports are submitted	The program's Medicaid Service Unit; abuse must also be reported to APS.[b]
Investigating	
Who is responsible for assessing incidents and conducting investigations	The Medicaid Service Unit is responsible for initial assessments and investigations.
How incidents are assessed	Reports are assessed and prioritized for investigation according to state criteria, and reports categorized as abuse, neglect, or exploitation are referred to APS.
Time frame for conducting and completing an investigation	APS investigations must be initiated within 3 working days, or, for emergency situations, within 4 hours. Findings must be submitted within 30 days to the District Attorney.
Notifying	
Process for informing the participant, or the participant's family or legal representative and other relevant parties, of the investigation results	Participant: must receive a copy of APS investigative findings. Family or legal representative: next of kin, caretakers, or legal guardians must receive a copy of the APS findings. Licensing and regulatory agency: must receive a copy of the APS findings.

Source: GAO analysis of the Centers for Diseases Control & Prevention data and the Centers for Medicare & Medicaid Services (CMS) HCBS waiver technical guidance and Oklahoma's waiver agreement. | GAO-19-599

[a] Medicaid made payments for 6 percent of assisted living residents in Oklahoma in 2014.

[b] The Oklahoma waiver program's Conditions for Provider Participation specify that assisted living facilities are required to follow APS's process for reporting potential instances of suspected abuse, neglect, or exploitation.

Figure 3. Oklahoma State Profile.

Numbers of Assisted Living Facilities, Licensed Beds, and Residents Financed by Medicaid Dollars, 2014			
State	Number of facilities	Number of beds	Number of residents financed by Medicaid
South Dakota	100	4,600	1,032[a]

Selected Mandatory Reporter Requirements

Reporting

Reporters—including assisted living facility staff—with cause to suspect abuse or neglect must notify the person in charge within 24 hours. Facility administrators must make an oral or written report within 24 hours to specified authorities, including South Dakota's Department of Human Services' Adult Protective Service (APS) program or law enforcement.

Investigating

No time frames for initiating or completing investigations are specified.

Notifying

No requirement to notify law enforcement. No requirement to notify family or legal guardian.

Home and Community-based Services (HCBS) Waiver Program Requirements

CMS waiver requires states specify	South Dakota's HCBS program requirements
Reporting	
Which types of incidents must be reported	Abuse, neglect, or exploitation along with other incidents such as a serious injury, death, missing person, or the provider's use of restraints or seclusion must be reported.
Who must report incidents	Providers contracted to provide waiver services are required to report incidents.
Time frames for reporting incidents	Serious injuries or suspected crimes must be reported within 2 hours, and other injuries within 24 hours.
To whom reports are submitted	Reports must be made to the Department of Human Services. Assisted living facilities must also submit critical incident reports to the facility's licensing and regulatory agency. Suspected crime must be reported to local law enforcement.
Investigating	
Who is responsible for assessing incidents and conducting investigations	The Department of Human Services is responsible for assessing and referring incidents as needed. State's attorney and law enforcement agencies must notify the Department of all reports they receive. The three entities work together on reports.
How incidents are assessed	Reports are categorized according to whether the report involves life- or health-threatening conditions or criminal activity, including suspected abuse.
Time frame for conducting and completing an investigation	For life- or health-threatening conditions or criminal activity, the Department of Human Services must make face-to-face contact within 24 hours. For other reports, they must make contact within 72 hours and face-to-face contact within 7 business days.
Notifying	
Process for informing the participant, or the participant's family or legal representative and other relevant parties, of the investigation results	Law enforcement: law enforcement must be notified by the Department of Human Services of reports of life- or health-threatening conditions or criminal activity, including abuse. Participant: no notification requirements are specified in the waiver agreement. Family or legal representative: no notification requirements in the waiver agreement. Licensing and regulatory agency: the Department of Health is notified of all incidents in facilities licensed by the Department of Health, and investigations are coordinated with Department of Health staff.

Source: GAO analysis of the Centers for Diseases Control & Prevention data and the Centers for Medicare & Medicaid Services (CMS) HCBS waiver technical guidance and South Dakota's waiver agreement. | GAO-19-599

[a] Medicaid made payments for 24 percent of assisted living residents in South Dakota in 2014.

Figure 4. South Dakota State Profile.

APPENDIX II: SUMMARY OF SELECTED FEDERAL AND STATE AUDITS OF OVERSIGHT OF THE REPORTING, INVESTIGATION, AND NOTIFICATION OF LAW ENFORCEMENT ABOUT ELDER ABUSE IN NURSING HOMES AND ASSISTED LIVING FACILITIES

GAO has issued reports reviewing the Centers for Medicare & Medicaid Services' (CMS) oversight of the health and welfare of residents in nursing homes and assisted living facilities.

Table 1. Examples of GAO Reports Relevant to Reporting and Investigation of Elder Abuse in Nursing Homes and Assisted Living Facilities, 2015-June 2019

Date	Title	Description
June 2019	Nursing Homes: Improved Oversight Needed to Better Protect Residents from Abuse (GAO-19-433)	GAO examined trends and types of abuse in nursing homes in recent years and CMS's oversight. GAO found that, while relatively rare, incidents of abuse as identified by state survey agencies more than doubled from 2013 to 2017, and that gaps in CMS oversight resulted in delays prioritizing investigations and notifying law enforcement about abuse. GAO made six recommendations including that CMS require state survey agencies to immediately notify law enforcement of any suspicion of a crime. HHS agreed with the recommendations and GAO will continue to monitor actions in response to the recommendations Setting: nursing homes
April 2019	Management Report: CMS Needs to Address Gaps in Federal Oversight of Nursing Home Abuse Investigations That Persisted in Oregon for at Least 15 Years (GAO-19-313R)	GAO reviewed CMS oversight of the Oregon state survey agency's investigation of complaints and facility-reported incidents of abuse in nursing homes in Oregon. GAO found that the Oregon survey agency was not following federal requirements that the survey agency investigate all abuse allegations in nursing homes. GAO made three recommendations including that CMS ensure all state survey agencies are meeting federal requirements for investigating alleged abuse and that the results are shared with CMS. HHS agreed with the recommendations and GAO will continue to monitor actions in response to the recommendations. Setting: nursing homes
January 2018	Medicaid Assisted Living Services: Improved Federal Oversight of Beneficiary Health and Welfare is Needed (GAO-18-179)	GAO examined state and federal oversight of assisted living services in Medicaid. GAO found oversight of state monitoring of assisted living services by CMS was limited by gaps in state reporting. GAO made three recommendations including that CMS clarify state requirements for reporting program deficiencies and require states to annually report critical incidents. HHS agreed with GAO's recommendations to clarify deficiency reporting and stated that it would consider annual reporting requirements for critical incidents after completing an ongoing review. As of June 2019, the recommendations remain open. Setting: assisted living facilities
August 2017	Medicaid Managed Care: CMS Should Improve Oversight of Access and Quality in States' Long-Term Services and Supports Programs (GAO-17-632)	GAO reviewed states' implementation and CMS's oversight of managed long-term services and supports programs. GAO found that states varied in the extent to which—and how—they monitored concerns about quality and access and CMS did not always require states to report the information needed to monitor access and quality. GAO made one recommendation that CMS take steps to identify and obtain information to oversee key aspects of managed long-term services and supports programs' access and quality, including network adequacy, critical incidents, and appeals and grievances. HHS agreed with GAO's recommendation. As of June 2019, the recommendation remains open. Setting: nursing homes, assisted living facilities, and others
October 2015	Nursing Home Quality: CMS Should Continue to Improve Data and Oversight (GAO-16-33)	GAO reviewed trends in nursing home quality data—including data on complaints and health and welfare deficiencies—and changes in CMS nursing home oversight. GAO found that trends in nursing home quality show mixed results (with data issues complicating the ability to assess quality trends) and that CMS made numerous modifications to its nursing home oversight activities, but has not monitored the potential effect of these modifications on nursing home quality oversight. GAO made three recommendations including that CMS implement a clear plan for ongoing auditing of self-reported data and establish a process for monitoring oversight modifications to better assess their effects. HHS agreed with GAO's recommendations. As of June 2019, one of the recommendations has been closed as implemented. Setting: nursing homes

Source: GAO. | GAO-19-599

Table 2. Examples of the Department of Health and Human Services, Office of Inspector General (HHS-OIG) Reports on the Reporting and Investigation of Elder Abuse in Nursing Homes, 2014-2018

Date	Title	Description
September 2017	HHS OIG Data Brief – A Few States Fell Short In Timely Investigation of the Most Serious Nursing Home Complaints: 2011-2015 (OEI-01-16-00330)	HHS-OIG reviewed nursing home complaints from 2011 through 2015 to identify the extent to which state survey agencies met onsite investigation timeframes for the most serious complaints. Key findings included: (1) states received one-third more reports of complaints in 2015 than in 2011 and (2) almost all states conducted onsite investigations within required timeframes. No specific recommendations were made. Setting: nursing homes
August 2017	Early Alert: The Centers for Medicare & Medicaid Services Has Inadequate Procedures to Ensure That Incidents of Potential Abuse or Neglect at Skilled Nursing Facilities Are Identified and Reported in Accordance With Applicable Requirements (A-01-17-00504)	HHS-OIG released the early alert as part of then-ongoing audits and investigations of nursing homes' performance in detecting and reporting elder abuse. Specifically, the audits are looking at whether incidents of potential abuse or neglect were reported and investigated in accordance with state and federal requirements. HHS-OIG found that a significant percentage of these incidents may not have been reported to law enforcement and that CMS has inadequate procedures to ensure that incidents of potential abuse or neglect of Medicare beneficiaries residing in nursing homes are identified and reported. In the agency's subsequent June 2019 report, HHS-OIG confirmed these findings and made a number of recommendations to CMS to provide training and clarify guidance for state survey agencies and nursing homes and track referrals to law enforcement.[a] CMS agreed with the recommendations. Setting: nursing homes
August 2014	Nursing Facilities' Compliance with Federal Regulations for Reporting Allegations of Abuse or Neglect (OEI-07-13-00010)	HHS-OIG examined the extent to which nursing homes reported allegations of abuse and neglect in 2012 and had policies in place for notifying law enforcement. Key findings included: (1) 85 percent of surveyed nursing homes reported at least one allegation of abuse or neglect in 2012 and (2) 76 percent of nursing homes had policies to address federal regulations for reporting and investigation of abuse or neglect. HHS-OIG made three recommendations regarding the reporting of abuse; CMS concurred with the recommendations. Setting: nursing homes

Source: GAO analysis of HHS-OIG reports. | GAO-19-599

[a] HHS-OIG. *Incidents of Potential Abuse and Neglect at Skilled Nursing Facilities Were Not Always Reported and Investigated.* A-01-16-00509 (Washington, D.C.: June 2019).

For example, selected GAO reports from approximately the past 5 years included a review of the incidence of abuse in nursing homes and a review of what is known about the incidence of abuse in assisted living facilities. Reports often included key recommendations. (See Table 1.)

In addition to GAO's audits of federal oversight of nursing homes and assisted living facilities, the Office of Inspector General within the Department of Health and Human Services (HHS-OIG) routinely audits a broad range of both the Centers for Medicare & Medicaid Services' (CMS) and states' oversight activities related to long-term care facilities.

We identified three HHS-OIG reports issued between 2014 and 2018 that provide examples of HHS-OIG's examinations of the reporting, investigation, and notification of law enforcement of elder abuse in nursing homes.[30] (See Table 2.) Although the specific scope of these reports varied, common findings included gaps in notifying law enforcement. For example, HHS-OIG examined Medicare claims data to identify cases where hospital staff had identified potential abuse and found that nursing homes failed to report many of these incidents to state survey agencies or notify law enforcement despite federal and state requirements and recommended that CMS provide training, clarify guidance, and track referrals to law enforcement.

State auditors may also audit their states' oversight of nursing homes and assisted living facilities. We identified nine reports issued by state auditors between 2014 and 2018 that examined their states' oversight of elder abuse reporting and investigation across both settings. (See Table 3.) Although the scope of individual reports across the states varied, state auditors identified instances of state entities not complying with state or federal requirements for a variety of reasons—including weaknesses in policies and procedures, resource constraints, and information management challenges—and recommended improvements. For example, in 2014 California state auditors found that thousands of complaint investigations—including over 300 classified as immediate jeopardy—were left open for almost a year, in part because the state did not specify time frames for completing investigations.

---

30 HHS-OIG officials told us that their agency has not reported on elder abuse in assisted living facilities specifically, but some of the agency's findings in other settings—e.g., group homes—may also apply to assisted living facilities.

Table 3. Examples of State Audit Reports on the Reporting and Investigation of Elder Abuse in Nursing Homes and Assisted Living Facilities, 2014-2018

State	Title	Source	Description
California	California Department of Public Health: It Has Not Effectively Managed Investigations of Complaints Related to Long-Term Health Care Facilities	California State Auditor (Oct. 2014)	The state auditor examined the state's Department of Public Health—which licenses and inspects nursing homes— compliance with state and federal requirements for the timeliness and quality of complaint investigations. Key findings included: (1) inadequate oversight of complaint processing and (2) lack of established investigation policies. The state auditor made a number of recommendations including specifying timeframes and developing policies for monitoring complaint processing and investigation. The Department did not agree with all the recommendations. Setting: nursing homes
Massachusetts	Executive Office of Elder Affairs (EOEA) Performance Audit	Office of the State Auditor, Massachusetts (2018)	The state auditor examined EOEA's process for screening, investigating, documenting and reporting incidents of elder abuse. The EOEA serves as the state's adult protective service (APS) and is responsible for investigating elder abuse in community settings including assisted living facilities. Key findings included: (1) a lack of reporting of abuse to investigative authorities; (2) a lack of documentation; and (3) weaknesses in monitoring of abuse report decisions. The state auditor made a number of recommendations including that EOEA develop written policies for documentation and review. EOEA agreed to implement the recommendations. Setting: assisted living facilities
Michigan	Follow-Up Report on Prior Audit Recommendations: Adult Protective Services (APS), Michigan Department of Health and Human Services	Office of the Auditor General, Michigan (2016)	The state auditor conducted a follow-up examination on a 2014 performance audit to determine whether APS had taken appropriate corrective action in response to previous findings. Among other things, these findings were related to compliance with the state's timeliness standards for investigations. The state auditor noted improvements but found that APS had not fully complied with earlier recommendations, and, as a result, investigations were not consistently initiated within required timeframes. The state auditor reiterated earlier recommendations; APS concurred. Setting: nursing homes and assisted living facilities
Minnesota	Office of Health Facility Complaints (OHFC) 2018 Evaluation Report	Office of the Legislative Auditor, Minnesota, (2018)	The state legislative auditor reviewed OHFC's ability to investigate allegations, impose enforcement measures, and communicate with complainants and stakeholders regarding their cases. Key findings included: (1) a lack of written policies, (2) information management system deficiencies, and (3) gaps in the state's regulatory structure resulting in less oversight of assisted living facilities than nursing homes. The legislative auditor made recommendations including legislative changes to improve accountability and oversight across facility types; OHFC largely concurred with the recommendations. Setting: nursing homes and assisted living facilities

State	Title	Source	Description
New Hampshire	State of New Hampshire Department of Health and Human Services Health Facility Licensing Unit (HFLU) Performance Audit Report	Office of the Legislative Budget Assistant, New Hampshire (2014)	The state legislative auditor examined the extent to which HFLU efficiently and effectively conducted inspections and complaint investigations in assisted living facilities and noncertified (i.e., private pay) nursing facilities. Key findings included a lack of policies and procedures. The auditor made several recommendations; HFLU agreed. Setting: assisted living facilities
New York	Department of Health Nursing Home Surveillance	Office of the State Comptroller, New York (2016)	The state auditor examined the extent to which the Department applied federal and state procedures for conducting nursing home surveys, and whether enforcement actions were effective in improving nursing home quality of care and safety. Key findings included that the state was generally meeting federal and state requirements, but that inefficient processes delayed enforcement actions. The state auditor recommended further action; the Department acknowledged the recommendations and noted actions underway. Setting: nursing homes
Ohio	Ohio Department of Health (ODH) Performance Audit Auditor of State,	Ohio (2017)	The state auditor reviewed and assessed selected program areas within ODH such as the Bureau of Long-Term Care and its processes to license, certify, and investigate complaints against long term care facilities. Key findings included identifying that staffing constraints contributed to inefficiencies during surveys and complaint investigations. The state auditor recommended diversifying hiring practices; ODH concurred. Setting: nursing homes and assisted living facilities
Pennsylvania	Performance Audit of the Department of Health (DOH)	Department of the Auditor General, Pennsylvania (2016)	The state auditor reviewed DOH's regulation of nursing homes, including a review of its policies and procedures for ensuring the quality of care provided, the effectiveness and timeliness of the agency's complaint response, and the consistency of its enforcement actions. Key findings included policy weaknesses that led to challenges in the states' ability to promptly investigate all incoming complaints. The state auditor made several recommendations including revised policies and procedures; DOH concurred. Setting: nursing homes
Washington	Performance Audit Complaint Resolution Unit (CRU) at the Department of Social and Health Services	Washington State Auditor (2015)	The state auditor examined whether CRU accurately prioritized and processed incoming complaint allegations from vulnerable adults in nursing homes and assisted living facilities on a timely basis. Key findings included: (1) an inefficient voicemail system that led to delays in investigations; (2) a lack of clarity in state law for required timeframes; and (3) inconsistent application of policy. The state auditor made several recommendations; CRU concurred. Setting: nursing homes and assisted living facilities

Source: GAO analysis of state auditor reports.| GAO-19-599

APPENDIX III: COMMENTS FROM THE DEPARTMENT OF HEALTH & HUMAN SERVICES

DEPARTMENT OF HEALTH & HUMAN SERVICES

OFFICE OF THE SECRETARY

Assistant Secretary for Legislation
Washington, DC 20201

JUL 2 6 2019

John E. Dicken
Director, Health Care Team
U.S. Government Accountability Office
441 G Street NW
Washington, DC 20548

Dear Mr. Dicken:

Attached are comments on the U.S. Government Accountability Office's (GAO) report entitled, "*Elder Abuse: Federal Requirements Differ for Oversight in Nursing Homes and Assisted Living Facilities*" (GAO-19-599).

The Department appreciates the opportunity to review this report prior to publication.

Sincerely,

for [signature]

Sarah Arbes
Acting Assistant Secretary for Legislation

GENERAL COMMENTS FROM THE DEPARTMENT OF HEALTH & HUMAN SERVICES ON THE GOVERNMENT ACCOUNTABILITY OFFICE'S DRAFT REPORT ENTITLED – ELDER ABUSE: FEDERAL REQUIREMENTS DIFFER FOR OVERSIGHT IN NURSING HOMES AND ASSISTED LIVING FACILITIES (GAO-19-599)

The U.S. Department of Health and Human Services (HHS) appreciates the opportunity to review and comment on the U.S. Government Accountability Office (GAO) draft report on federal oversight of elder abuse reporting, investigation, and law enforcement notification. Every resident deserves to be treated with dignity and kept safe from abuse and neglect. Resident safety in facilities that participate in the Medicare and Medicaid programs is a top priority for HHS.

Regardless of facility type, HHS is committed to ensuring the safety of residents and directly overseeing and supporting states' oversight of reporting, investigating, and notifying law enforcement about elder abuse. In this report, GAO directly compared federal oversight requirements of nursing homes receiving Medicare and Medicaid payments and assisted living facilities providing services to Medicaid beneficiaries. As GAO reported, only 16.5 percent of assisted living facilities use Medicaid as a payer source. It is important to note that HHS oversees these facilities in partnership with states that have received a Medicaid home and community-based service (HCBS) waiver, also known as a 1915(c) waiver, or a 1915(i) Medicaid State Plan Amendment (SPA) to provide assisted living facility services to Medicaid beneficiaries. In contrast, HHS has direct oversight responsibility over nursing homes. Therefore, these two types of federal oversight are not directly comparable.

Although HHS' oversight of assisted living facilities is limited to states' HCBS waivers and SPAs that may provide assisted living facilities services for Medicaid beneficiaries, HHS is engaged in supporting states in overseeing these facilities and ensuring the safety of beneficiaries. In an effort to strengthen community living options for older Americans and people with disabilities, HHS issued a final rule in 2014[1] that set forth requirements for several Medicaid authorities under which states may provide home and community-based services. In particular, as part of the 1915(c) waiver approval process, each waiver must have a Quality Improvement Strategy wherein the state demonstrates that it has designed and implemented an effective system for assuring participant health and welfare. As part of this system, HHS requires states to develop and measure performance indicators in fourteen areas, which are reported to HHS in the form of an annual report. In addition, the annual report to HHS must include a mandatory quality improvement project/remediation when the compliance threshold for a performance measure is below 86 percent.[2]

HHS also offers technical assistance resources to states to improve quality under HCBS programs. This includes a 2014 Informational Bulletin that modifies the quality assurance systems under 1915(c) waivers to strengthen the oversight of beneficiary health and welfare reporting requirements.[3] Specifically, this guidance modified HHS requirements regarding reporting on individual remediation, requiring states to report on individual activities related to instances of substantiated abuse, neglect and/or exploitation. Furthermore, in January 2015, HHS

[1] 79 FR 2948

[2] https://www.medicaid.gov/medicaid-chip-program-information/by-topics/waivers/downloads/3-cmcs-quality-memo-narrative.pdf

[3] https://www.medicaid.gov/medicaid-chip-program-information/by-topics/waivers/downloads/3-cmcs-quality-memo-narrative.pdf

updated a 1915(c) technical guide, which outlines HHS' expectations on what states need to include in their waiver application with regard to reporting and investigating critical events or incidents.[4] Lastly, HHS provides monthly webinars to states on a variety of HCBS topics. For example, in January 2017, HHS conducted a webinar to assist states in creating and implementing quality and performance measures across the HCBS authorities, including a focus on remediation reporting requirements.

HHS works in partnership with state survey agencies to oversee nursing homes, since these agencies are generally responsible for state licensure. The state survey agencies visit and survey every Medicare and Medicaid participating nursing home in the nation at least annually to ensure they are meeting CMS' health and safety requirements as well as state licensure requirements. For nursing homes, the state survey agencies not only inspect providers for compliance with Medicare and Medicaid health and safety standards, but also manage the intake of complaints and facility-reported incidents and conduct investigations accordingly. Residents deserve consistent nursing home quality, regardless of location, so HHS is revising its oversight of state survey agency performance. HHS is examining the way surveyors identify issues such as abuse, facility staffing levels, and dementia care, and is clarifying expectations regarding when abuse must be reported to the state and law enforcement. This means setting clear timelines for state survey agencies to review allegations of abuse and neglect.

HHS' approach to oversight of nursing homes is constantly evolving, and we're continuously looking for ways to improve our approach to nursing home safety and quality. HHS is undertaking a comprehensive review of our regulations, guidelines, internal structure, and processes related to safety and quality in nursing homes. HHS has demonstrated a commitment to this path by developing a five-part plan to ensure the care provided in nursing homes is of the highest possible quality. The five-part plan will strengthen oversight, enhance enforcement, increase transparency, improve quality, and put patients over paperwork.[5]

In addition to HHS efforts to strengthen federal oversight of nursing homes and states with HCBS programs, CMS has committed to addressing numerous recommendations from GAO and OIG to further strengthen reporting, investigating, and notifying law enforcement about elder abuse.

---

[4] https://wms-mmdl.cms.gov/WMS/faces/portal.jsp

[5] https://www.cms.gov/blog/ensuring-safety-and-quality-americas-nursing-homes

INDEX

A

B

C

D

E

F

G

H

I

L

M

N

O

P

Q

R

S

T

U

V

W

Y